Managing Childbirth Emergencies in Community Settings

Edited by

Vivien Woodward,
Karen Bates
and
Nicki Young

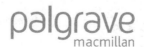

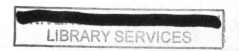

First published 2005 by
PALGRAVE MACMILLAN
Houndmills, Basingstoke, Hampshire RG21 6XS and
175 Fifth Avenue, New York, N.Y. 10010
Companies and representatives throughout the world

PALGRAVE MACMILLAN is the global academic imprint of the Palgrave Macmillan division of St. Martin's Press, LLC and of Palgrave Macmillan Ltd. Macmillan® is a registered trademark in the United States, United Kingdom and other countries. Palgrave is a registered trademark in the European Union and other countries.

ISBN 1–4039–0517–7

This book is printed on paper suitable for recycling and made from fully managed and sustained forest sources.

A catalogue record for this book is available from the British Library.

10	9	8	7	6	5	4	3	2	1
14	13	12	11	10	09	08	07	06	05

Printed and bound in China

Contents

List of Figures and Tables

Figures

Tables

Acknowledgements

We wish to thank everyone who has contributed to the book and shared their knowledge and experience of managing childbirth emergencies. We thank Philip Ball, Senior Medical Artist, University of Cambridge, for providing original Figures 4.3, 6.1, 6.2, 7.2 and 7.3. Thanks also go to Maggie Bunting, Lorraine Skipper and Melinda Bird for reading and validating the problem-based scenario in Chapter 3. We are very appreciative of their time and suggestions.

We also wish to express our appreciation to the School of Nursing and Midwifery, University of East Anglia, Norwich, Norfolk, to Homerton College Cambridge, School of Health Studies, and to colleagues, friends and family who supported us through this work.

The publisher and authors would like to thank the organisations listed below for permission to reproduce material from their publications:

Elsevier Ltd for Figures 2.1, 2.2, 2.4, 2.5, 5.6, 6.3 and 6.4, from Betty Sweet et al., *Mayes Midwifery*, 12th edition, pp. 523, 527, 707 and 710, Copyright 1997; Figure 5.7 from D. James et al., *High Risk Pregnancy: Management Options*, 2nd edition, Copyright 1999; Figure 6.5 from Beischer, *Ostetrics and the Newborn: An Illustrated Textbook*, 2nd edition, Copyright 1986.

Radcliffe Medical Press Ltd for Figures 2.3, 4.2, 4.4 and 4.5 from M. Boyle, *Emergencies Around Childbirth: A Handbook for Midwives*, 2002.

The Resuscitation Council for Figures 7.2, 7.3, 7.4 and 7.5 from *Newborn Life Support Provider Course Manual 2001*.

Every effort has been made to obtain necessary permission with reference to copyright material. The publisher and authors apologise if, inadvertently, any sources remain unacknowledged and will be glad to make the necessary arrangements at the earliest opportunity.

Vivien Woodward
Karen Bates
Nicki Young

List of Contributors

Hamid Al-Taher MBBCH, MSc, MOG Liverpool, FRCOG is Consultant Obstetrician and Gynaecologist and Clinician Manager of the Women and Children Directorate in the Queen Elizabeth NHS Hospital Trust, Kings Lynn, Norfolk where he has worked for 11 years.

Karen Bates MA, DPSM, RM, RN is Midwifery Lecturer and Course Director for Midwifery Post-registration Studies at the School of Nursing and Midwifery, University of East Anglia, Norwich. She has a particular interest in the midwifery management of emergencies during childbirth and undertakes expert witness work in all areas of midwifery practice, but particularly in relation to shoulder dystocia. Karen's midwifery experience includes leading a team of midwives providing 24-hour integrated midwifery care. This included intrapartum care in the home as well as in hospital.

Glenys Boxwell BSc (Hons), RN, RSCN, ENB 400, Cert Ed. is Clinical Nurse Leader on the NICU Addenbrookes NHS Hospital Trust, Cambridge, and has been a neonatal intensive care nurse and lecturer in neonatal care since 1985. She has also been a newborn life support instructor for many years. Previous publications include *Neonatal Intensive Care Nursing* published by Routledge in 2000.

Maggie Bunting DPSM, RM, RN is a practice development midwife at the Norfolk and Norwich University Hospital NHS Trust, Norwich. She has 14 years' experience as a midwife, including six years working as part of an integrated team providing care in community and hospital settings, which included a home birth rate of one to two per month.

Stuart Brown BSC (Hons), MBChB, FRCA is currently a specialist registrar in anaesthesia at Addenbrookes' NHS Hospital Trust, Cambridge, England.

Susan Burvill MSc, BSc (Hons), RM, RN is a consultant midwife at the Rosie Hospital, Cambridge. Previous to this post Susan worked in education and for several years as an independent midwife. She has also worked abroad in other European countries, the former Soviet Union bloc and the developing world.

Ann Compton RM, RN has many years' experience as a community midwife and supervisor of midwives. More recently she has been practising as a clinical midwife and midwifery manager in Norfolk.

Kenda Crozier MSc, BSc, RM, RN, PGDipHE is a lecturer in midwifery at the University of East Anglia and her research interests include interprofessional education and technology in midwifery.

Pat Lindsay MSc (Medical Sociology), ADM, PGCEA, RM, RN is a midwife at the Rosie Hospital, Cambridge, responsible for maternity care assistant training. She has been involved in midwifery education and practice for many years, which included work in a stand-alone GP unit, equivalent to a midwifery-led unit. Her publications include chapters for *Mayes' Midwifery* (12th edition) and a number of journal articles.

John Scott MB, ChB, DA, DobsRCOG, DFFP, FIMC, RCS(Ed) is Clinical Director of the East Anglian Ambulance NHS Trust, Norwich. He has a particular interest in the practice of and education in pre-hospital emergency care.

Natasha Taylor SRP is a paramedic in the East Anglian Ambulance NHS Trust and presently attached to the Clinical Directorate as a clinical instructor.

Amanda Williamson LLM, LLB (Hons), RM, RGN, ACHEP is a lecturer in midwifery at the University of East Anglia and has a particular interest in the law in relation to health care practice but in particular the law relating to children.

Vivien Woodward PhD, MSC, PGCEA, MTD, ADM, RM, RN, is Senior Midwifery Lecturer at Homerton College, Cambridge, School of Health Studies, and has worked as a midwife since the 1970s. This included practice as a community midwife attached to a GP unit in Suffolk. During the past 16 years she has worked in midwifery education and research. Her PhD was based on an ethnographic study to explore the meaning and practice of professional caring in nursing and midwifery settings and she has published articles on a variety of midwifery-associated topics.

Nicki Young MSc, RM, RN, PGDipHE is a lecturer in midwifery at the University of East Anglia. Her research interests include clinical decision-making in midwifery and the midwifery care received by women who undergo termination of pregnancy for fetal abnormality. As part-requirement of a Doctorate in Education programme, she is currently undertaking an ethnographic study to explore how direct entry student midwives develop clinical decision-making skills.

1

Introduction: Setting the Context of the Book

Vivien Woodward

The inspiration

This book was inspired by an interest and commitment that my fellow co-editors, Karen Bates and Nicki Young, and I shared in our work as midwifery lecturers preparing both student and qualified midwives to manage emergencies in the absence of immediate obstetric assistance. From the discussions of our individual experiences we identified two concerns: first, there appeared to be an in-built assumption by many students and midwives that obstetric intervention would be immediately available. This suggested a limited awareness of the possibility that a woman's and/or her infant's life might ultimately lie in their hands. For example, when we presented students or midwives with scenarios where an emergency had occurred in the home, or the consultant unit obstetrician was busy in theatre and was unable to attend, some were hesitant about what they would do after their initial actions and lacked knowledge about subsequent emergency procedures and manoeuvres. Some questioned if they could or even should undertake them. In particular, the requirement to undertake the procedure of manual removal of placenta in the management of severe primary postpartum haemorrhage (UKCC 1998) provoked intense anxiety.

Secondly, we shared a frustration. As we sought evidence and guidance to support our teaching, we established that information about the midwife's management of childbirth emergencies in community settings is virtually non-existent. Of the many midwifery, labour ward and

1

obstetric textbooks reviewed, all reflect the assumption that immediate obstetric help is available.

As the following paragraphs explain, there has been a significant shift in the philosophical aims of the maternity services during the past decade. Midwives have expanded their community-based services substantially in response to women's desire for minimal intervention and maximum satisfaction. As a result, midwives' management of emergencies in the community and working partnership with other maternity care professionals have become critical issues which need urgently to be addressed.

The increase in community-based intrapartum care

The Changing Childbirth Report (DoH 1993) emphasised and legitimated the importance of the social, emotional and spiritual aspects of childbirth which, until then, had become subsumed by the medical model of care during the previous three decades (Bryar 1995). In practice, this new philosophy means giving women evidence-based information about care options, as well as facilitating their individual wishes (Page 2000) and empowering them to decline unwanted routine obstetric interventions. In this way, women are enabled to achieve a satisfying and meaningful, as well as safe, childbirth experience. In particular, the report advocated genuine choice for women regarding the place of birth and endorsed this based on evidence that hospital birth does not provide any added benefits in low-risk cases. This pronouncement was an important milestone in the evolution of maternity care in the UK and set an official precedent for challenging established medical authority. It brought about a brave new world, in which women and midwives, in partnership, were empowered to reject practices based merely on tradition, authority and myth and to prioritise choice above compliance.

In response to the Changing Childbirth Report recommendations, the rate of home birth in the UK increased from almost 1 per cent of births in 1987 to 2.6 per cent in 2003 (Phipps 2003), and is forecast to rise to 4 or 5 per cent by 2005 (Chamberlain et al. 1999). Because of the possibility of unanticipated emergencies, it is acknowledged that midwives accept immense responsibility when undertaking planned home births (DoH 1993). Indeed, it was recognised that the report (DoH 1993) initiated a time of major transition for midwives. Midwifery clinical skills and confidence, eroded as a result of the deeply embedded hospital model of maternity care, had to be regained to enable midwives working in the National Health Service to take on the responsibility of home births and the lead professional role (SNMAC 1998). Ten years on, our observations mentioned at the beginning of the chapter, supported by a number of studies identifying midwives' lack of confidence in managing home births (Phipps 2003, Galloway 1995, Hosein 1998) and high-risk situations (Hosein 1998, Pope et al. 1996), indicate that the transition is still in progress.

Whether as a result of safety issues or organisational factors (Phipps 2003, Hosein 1998, Galloway 1995), ambivalent attitudes towards home birth may account for the rapid growth in popularity of midwifery-led birth centres which aim to provide non-interventionist care in a 'home-from-home setting' (Tinsley 2003, p. 14). Whilst some of the centres are integrated within consultant units, others are based in the community and may be some distance from the hospital. Although birth centres may be perceived as a safer alternative to home birth, it is crucial that, whatever the birth setting, midwives are alert to the possibility of unanticipated complications and emergencies, and can manage them and procure medical assistance as soon as possible in accordance with the statutory framework (UKCC 1998).

The increase in community-based intrapartum care goes hand in hand with the current midwifery discourse of redefining and promoting 'normal childbirth' (RCM 2000). The movement aims to eradicate the unwarranted obstetric intervention associated with the pathologising perspective that childbirth is only 'normal in retrospect' (Murphy-Lawless 1998) which has pervaded the maternity services for many years. However, whilst acknowledging the need to avoid unnecessary medical intervention, Hodnett (2003) suggests that an overemphasis on normality may adversely affect caregivers' ability to detect, act upon or acquire assistance with complications. Midwives are in a position to make a significant contribution to women's health and wellbeing by recognising, responding to and referring childbirth complications and emergencies promptly and effectively, and are being urged to develop this aspect of practice (NICE 2001). This responsibility not only relates to planned home birth and care in midwifery-led birth centres but also to the need to address the poor outcomes experienced by the substantial number of women who deliver unexpectedly at home (Young 1999). It is essential that the midwifery profession should not only guard normal childbirth and minimise unnecessary obstetric intervention but also promote the on-going development of midwives' contribution to reducing morbidity and mortality in emergency and high-risk situations.

Hospital midwives

Whilst this book focuses on community-based midwifery practice, it is also relevant to hospital-based midwives, whether in consultant or integrated midwifery-led units. Although midwives may anticipate that obstetric help will be readily available, professional and organisational changes increase the onus on midwives to detect complications and manage emergencies in hospital settings as in the community. In particular, there are concerns regarding medical staffing levels on labour wards as a result of the reduction of junior doctors' hours and reduced experience requirements involved in specialist registrar training (RCOG/RCM 1999). These factors combine to place greater demands on obstetric consultants whose numbers remain relatively unchanged. A strategy put forward to manage this medical staffing shortfall is to have a clear demarcation of roles, albeit within the context of close multiprofessional teamworking. Midwives are responsible for women in normal labour and have a senior midwife for advice and support, whilst medical staff are responsible for women with complicated labours or complex obstetric problems. As previously mentioned, unexpected emergencies occur and midwives need to consider the implications the RCOG/RCM (1999) guidelines. These recommend that a doctor of at least 12 months' experience should always be available to attend emergencies within five minutes, and a doctor with at least three years' experience within 30 minutes. A woman's condition could deteriorate rapidly within these timeframes and, should there be delay, hospital midwives, like their community counterparts, need to have their action plans prepared. For example, in the case of primary postpartum haemorrhage, if they have rubbed up a contraction, given the permitted doses of oxytocic, and emptied the bladder and uterus, what they would do next, faced with a woman with torrential bleeding?

The rationale for the book

A decade has passed since the publication of the Changing Childbirth Report (DoH 1993) stimulated a substantial increase in community-based midwifery services and encouraged midwives to take on more responsibility and to fulfil the potential of their role. But there still remains a lack of both clinical and professional guidance for managing high-risk situations and childbirth emergencies 'in the field'. This book aims to start the process of addressing this deficit.

Midwives are most likely to be the first health professionals at the sharp end of childbirth emergencies in the community but certainly not the only ones. It is important to develop a working partnership with paramedics and/or GPs who may also, on occasion, be first on the scene. It is hoped, therefore, that all three professional groups will find the book informative and of practical help and that it will stimulate reflective and collaborative practice.

The structure of the book

Chapters 2 to 7 have a clinical focus and cover the major high-risk situations and/or childbirth emergencies. Each chapter provides the relevant physiology and pathophysiology which underpins clinical assessment and subsequent decision-making, and a step-by-step guide of the management of the situation in the absence of obstetric and/or paediatric assistance. When and how to deal with the emergency in situ, factors contributing to the decision to transfer into hospital, preparations for transfer, and care during transfer are also discussed. Psychosocial issues specific to the emergency are outlined in order to promote a holistic approach to care.

The remaining chapters address professional issues. Chapter 8 provides an account of the role of the paramedic service, about which little has previously been published, despite this being the profession most often called to assist in emergency situations in the community and the vital importance of understanding one another's roles as part of effective teamworking. Chapter 9 aims to support midwives in their goal to increase women's childbirth options by exploring a number of important professional and legal issues with which midwives need to be cognisant in order to practice safely and accountably. Chapter 10 identifies strategies within midwifery pre- and post-registration programmes to prepare students/midwives to act effectively when faced with childbirth emergencies. The impact of the tensions between midwives and medical staff on clinical care and the potential of shared education to help address the problem are examined in Chapter 11.

Commentaries by supervisor of midwives

Promoting choice and normality in childbirth creates grey areas in practice and makes midwifery supervision a vital safeguard not only for women and their families but also for midwives. For example, in adopting the social model of maternity care, midwives are called to enable women to 'achieve the outcome the woman believes is best for her baby and herself' (DoH 1993 p. 25). Midwives may find themselves supporting women to have home birth against obstetric advice and/or established research evidence (Page 2000). A commentary by a supervisor of midwives is included in Chapters 2 to 6 in order to provide additional professional guidance.

The purpose of the obstetric commentaries

Perhaps because of traditional hierarchical structures, health professionals tend to learn in isolation from one another (McFarlane and Downe 1999). Whilst the management of emergencies in the book is written from a midwifery perspective, it embraces a key philosophy in the Changing Childbirth Report (DoH 1993) that only through multiprofessional working is genuine, woman-centred care achievable. The report acknowledged the responsibility that midwives accept in caring for a woman who wishes to have a home birth and envisioned that consultant obstetricians would play a part in providing advice and support to midwives undertaking home births. For these reasons, a commentary by a consultant obstetrician is included in Chapters 2 to 6.

Problem-based scenarios and interactive action planning exercises

A problem-based scenario and interactive action planning exercise is placed at the end of each of the chapters dealing with a specific emergency (Chapters 2 to 6). These exercises aim to:

1   place the reader in the role of the professional taking responsibility for the situation enabling him or her mentally to rehearse and to formulate action plans;
2   consolidate learning by applying the information covered in the chapter to a clinical situation;
3   stimulate critical thinking and reasoning skills as the reader needs to give an account of his/her actions;
4   identify areas for further study/information-gathering.

Readers are strongly advised to read through the relevant chapter before attempting the action planning exercise, in order to get full details about the specific management of the emergency.

How to work through the exercises

- Read through the sequence of scenarios. After each scenario, you will be asked questions to explore your understanding of the situation and the actions you would take.
- Expect to spend about five to ten minutes answering each question.
- Go back through the chapter to check on any points that you are unsure about.
- Assess your learning by comparing your responses with the checklist of points in the boxes.
- Make a note of any gaps in your knowledge and further information you need to find out, for example local policies, procedures and contact details.
- Throughout the exercise consider if you would be able to justify your decisions and actions.
- You may find it beneficial to discuss the scenarios with a colleague.
- A model doll and pelvis will be helpful for some of the exercises.

References

Bryar, R (1995) *Theory for Midwifery Practice*. Macmillan: London.

Chamberlain, G, Wraight, A and Crowley, P (1999) Birth at Home; A Report of the National Survey of Home Births in the UK by the National Birthday Trust, *The Practising Midwife* **2** (7), 35–9.

DoH (Department of Health) (1993) *Changing Childbirth. The Report of the Expert Maternity Group. Part One*. HMSO: London.

Galloway, M (1995) GPs and Midwives Still Divided on Homebirths, *Modern Midwife* **5** (7), 7–9.

Hodnett, E D (2003) Home-like Versus Conventional Institutional Settings for Birth (Cochrane Review). In *The Cochrane Library*, Issue 3, Update Software: Oxford.

Hosein, M (1998) Home Birth: Is it a Real Option? *British Journal of Midwifery* **6** (6), 370–3.

McFarlane, S and Downe, S (1999) *Southern Derbyshire Training and Education Project for Maternity Services*. Southern Derbyshire Acute Hospital NHS Trust: Derby.

Murphy-Lawless, J (1998) *Reading Birth and Death. A History of Obstetric Thinking*. Cork University Press: Cork.

NICE (National Institute for Clinical Excellence) (2001) *Confidential Enquiries into Maternal Deaths (CEMD). (2001) Why Mothers Die 1997–1999.* NICE: London.

Page, L., (ed) (2000) *The New Midwifery. Science and Sensitivity in Practice.* Churchill Livingstone: London.

Phipps, B (2003) Homebirth: What Does it Mean to Women? In B Lee, Homebirth – A Realistic Possibility? *RCM Midwives* **6** (5), 204–7.

Pope, R, Cooney, M, Graham, L and Holliday, M (1996) *Identification of the Changing Educational Needs of Midwives in Developing New Dimensions of Care in a Variety of Settings and the Development of a Package to Meet these Needs.* English National Board for Nursing, Midwifery and Health Visiting: London.

RCM (Royal College of Midwives) (2000) *Vision 2000.* RCM: London.

RCOG/RCM (Royal College of Obstetricians and Gynaecologists) and (Royal College of Midwives (1999) *Towards Safer Childbirth. Minimum Standards for the Organisation of Labour Wards.* RCOG Press: London.

SNMAC (Standing Nursing and Midwifery Advisory Committee) (1998) *Midwifery: Delivering Our Future.* DoH: London.

Tinsley, V (2003) Birth Centres in Wiltshire (1). *The Practising Midwife* **6** (5), 14–20.

UKCC (United Kingdom Central Council for Nursing, Midwifery and Health Visiting) (1998) *The Midwives Rules and Code of Practice.* UKCC: London.

Young, G (1999) The Case for Community-Based Maternity Care. In G Marsh and M Renfrew (eds), *Community-Based Maternity Care.* Oxford University Press: Oxford.

2

Antepartum and Postpartum Haemorrhage in the Community

Maggie Bunting

Introduction

Haemorrhage is repeatedly an important cause of maternal death in the triennial reports of the CEMD (Confidential Enquiries into Maternal Deaths in the UK). Placental abruption, placenta praevia and postpartum haemorrhage are the main causes of severe haemorrhage that can result in maternal death. Maternal morbidity following obstetric haemorrhage includes hypovolaemic shock, disseminated intravascular coagulation (DIC), renal failure, hepatic failure, Sheehan's syndrome and anaemia. Haemorrhage in pregnancy also puts the fetus at significant risk of hypoxia and death in utero.

The aims of this chapter are to aid the prompt recognition and diagnosis of antepartum and postpartum haemorrhage and haemorrhagic shock and the immediate management of these situations in community settings, such as the home and non-integrated midwifery-led unit. Readers are referred to obstetric texts, for example Sweet (1997) for full information about management once in hospital.

Definitions

The definition of antepartum haemorrhage (APH) is bleeding from the genital tract after the 24th week of pregnancy. APH is often unpredictable and can become a life-threatening massive obstetric haemorrhage very quickly (Konje and Taylor 1999). At term maternal blood is circulating to the placenta at about 500 ml per minute. Consequently, blood loss may be rapid and devastating.

The definition of postpartum haemorrhage (PPH) is excessive bleeding from the genital tract from the birth of the baby to the end of the puerperium, either 500 ml or any amount sufficient to cause maternal cardiovascular compromise. If bleeding occurs within 24 hours it is called primary PPH. Secondary or 'late' PPH is defined as excessive vaginal bleeding between 24 hours and six weeks following delivery and is much less common.

It needs to be remembered that it can be difficult to estimate blood loss. When blood forms in a clot, its size reduces to 40 per cent and therefore the amount, when measured, should be doubled. Estimation of blood loss is complicated further in cases of placental abruption where massive bleeding may be concealed.

APH and PPH can lead to a torrential obstetric haemorrhage. There is no consensus on the definition of massive obstetric haemorrhage. Some experts believe that the crucial element is the amount of blood lost, while others focus on the amount of blood that needs to be replaced, as the following extracts suggest:

- 'When the patient's blood loss is over 1500 ml, which represents around 25 per cent of the blood volume' (Bonnar 2000).
- 'A replacement of 50 per cent of circulating blood volume in less than three hours of more than 150 ml per minute' (Sakhry and Sheldon 1994).
- 'Rapid transfusion of a substantial volume of fluid and red cell replacement is likely to be required over a few hours as a result of major bleeding that may prove difficult to control surgically' (McClelland 1995).

Notably, all these definitions only allow the diagnosis of haemorrhage to be established in hindsight. However, the management of obstetric haemorrhage requires immediate response; delay in instigating care is known to increase maternal and neonatal mortality and morbidity. In clinical midwifery and obstetric practice, response to any bleeding that is more than the norm, for the current real time situation, should be immediate. An analogous situation is shoulder dystocia where the more manoeuvres required to deliver the baby the more severe the shoulder dystocia. Any obstetric haemorrhage should be similarly viewed: the longer it takes to control the bleeding, the more severe the situation, regardless of the amount of blood loss.

A woman's general health and wellbeing will allow a variance in what blood loss can be suffered without adverse consequences. A healthy pregnant woman at term will tolerate up to 1000 ml blood loss with minimal signs and symptoms (Bonnar 2000). The increase in circulating blood volume that occurs in pregnancy, and a marked increase in coagulation factors, for example fibrinogen, factors VII and VIII, will offer the woman physiological protection against haemorrhage. However, if a pregnant woman has hypotension with a blood pressure below 80 mmHg, this will usually indicate a blood loss in excess of 1500 ml (Bonnar 2000). This degree of blood loss will lead to vasoconstriction in order to maintain perfusion of the maternal heart and brain at the expense of uteroplacental blood flow. Fetal compromise in such a situation is a further indication that the antepartum haemorrhage is substantial. Shock from any condition will inevitably cause progress to multi-organ failure and death unless some compensatory mechanisms occur to reverse the situation or clinical treatments are successful.

Antepartum haemorrhage

The incidence of antepartum haemorrhage is 2 to 5 per cent of all pregnancies (Green 1989). Approximately 50 per cent of vaginal bleeding in pregnancy remains indeterminate in its cause. It may be due to factors such as a 'show', bleeding from the cervix, trauma or genital infection but more commonly it is the result of marginal sinus rupture (Scott 1986). Such factors are often difficult to diagnose. There are two main classified causes of APH: placenta praevia and placental abruption.

Placenta praevia

The placenta normally embeds in the fundus in the upper uterine segment. Placenta praevia is a placenta that has embedded partially or wholly in the lower uterine segment. The location of the placenta in relation to the cervix classifies its grade (Figure 2.1). Type I the placenta is encroaching on the lower segment but does not reach the internal os; Type II the placenta reaches but does not cover the internal os; Type III

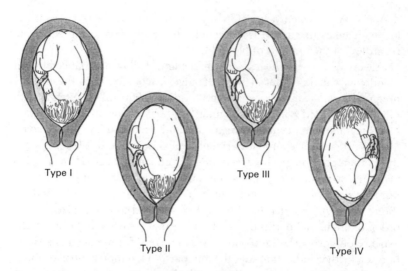

Type I

Type III

Type II

Type IV

Figure 2.1   Placenta praevia types I to IV

the placenta covers the internal os asymmetrically; Type IV the placenta symmetrically covers the internal os. Increased age, increased parity, previous history of placenta praevia and previous Caesarean section are associated with an increase risk of placenta praevia.

Placenta praevia carries with it the risk of maternal mortality due to haemorrhage. A key point made in CEMD (NICE 2001) was that placenta praevia, particularly in women with a previous uterine scar, may be associated with uncontrolled uterine haemorrhage at delivery and Caesarean hysterectomy may be necessary. The increased risk of haemorrhage postpartum is thought to be due to inadequate ability of the sinuses in the lower uterine segment to occlude maternal sinuses and control the bleeding. Placenta accreta occurs in 15 per cent of women with placenta praevia (Konje and Taylor 1999). The risk to the fetus include prematurity, intrauterine growth retardation, increased incidence of congenital malformations, malpresentation, cord prolapse, fetal anaemia and intrauterine death due to severe maternal haemorrhagic shock (Konje and Taylor 1999).

Ultrasound scans at 20 weeks' gestation can detect a low-lying placenta but, as the lower uterine segment has not formed at this stage, the diagnosis of placenta praevia cannot be made. A finding of a low-lying placenta is common in early pregnancy but as the upper uterine segment enlarges and the lower segments forms, the placental localisation will be above the lower uterine segment by 24 weeks in 82 per cent of cases (Hibbard 1988). The NICE guidelines on antenatal care (2003) recommend that if the placenta is found to extend across the internal os, another scan at 36 weeks should be offered. However, it is important to note in the community setting that even with an early scan showing a low-lying placenta (unless covering the os) no further scans may be arranged until there is a clinical indication.

Clinical presentation and management

Placenta praevia usually presents very characteristically. There is a history of painless bleeding as the blood from the site of placental detachment, which might otherwise infiltrate the myometrium and cause pain, escapes vaginally. For this reason the uterus will be soft on palpation. The vaginal bleeding has no evident cause, although it can be provoked during sexual intercourse. Bleeding due to placenta praevia commonly manifests itself between 34 and 36 weeks' gestation when development of the lower uterine segment causes cervical effacement and associated separation of the low-lying placenta (Lindsay 1997a). It is the absence of pain that is often used to distinguish placenta praevia from placental abruption.

However, 10 per cent of women with placenta praevia will have a coexisting abruption (Hibbard 1988), and women experiencing painful contractions may make diagnosis of placenta praevia a challenge. It is important to assess her for signs of pre-eclampsia in order to exclude a coexisting risk of placental abruption.

During abdominal palpation, the position of the placenta in the lower uterine segment will prevent the fetal presenting part engaging and can make a longitudinal lie impossible (Konje and Taylor 1999). Placenta praevia is therefore frequently associated with malpresentation, such as breech and transverse or oblique lie. ***Vaginal or rectal examinations must not be performed following an antepartum haemorrhage*** because, if the cause is placenta praevia, further haemorrhage may be provoked (Konje and Taylor 1999).

A woman who has already been diagnosed as having a low-lying placenta or placenta praevia will be very anxious, and even more so if haemorrhage occurs in a community setting. The establishment of a trusting relationship by any health professional attending is essential in order to provide optimum care and assistance.

There needs to be an initial assessment of the amount of blood loss by vulval inspection and counting the number of bloodstained pads or sheets (which should be saved in order to estimate the total blood loss). One ml of blood weighs one gram, and therefore weighing pads (which is possibly more accurately undertaken in the hospital) may help in the estimation. The amount comprising blood clots should be doubled. It is important for the midwife accurately to document the estimation in order to assist a paramedic/anaesthetist in making an assessment for fluid replacement.

Arrange immediate transfer to hospital

A woman with active vaginal bleeding needs to be transferred to a hospital with intensive care facilities, blood transfusion capabilities, theatres, and senior anaesthetic and obstetric cover. Urgent transfer should be arranged by paramedic ambulance.

In addition to calling for paramedic attendance, the midwife may, while waiting for the paramedics, summon further assistance from a second health professional, which will allow:

- assistance in resuscitation;
- the family to be supported;
- help in arranging urgent transfer to hospital.

Resuscitation, restoration of blood volume and transfer into hospital

Prior to and during transfer, the mother should be supported in lying on her left side to avoid postural hypotension. Oxygen at 10 litres per minute may be administered via face mask if there is concern about fetal compromise.

Maternal pulse and blood pressure need to be measured and recorded quarter-hourly to detect signs of shock indicated by a rising pulse rate, becoming thready, tachypnoea, reducing blood pressure, and being pale, clammy and restless. The mother may appear confused owing to hypoxia and, if the blood pressure reading is below her normal baseline measurement and the blood loss appears to be substantial, fluid replacement is essential.

Intravenous cannulation by the midwife, paramedic or GP at this stage may be easier to achieve before substantial peripheral shutdown occurs and will allow instant access as soon as intravenous fluid replacement is available. Two 14-gauge intravenous cannulae are required in an obstetric emergency and the use of a wide lumen intravenous giving set (a blood-giving set) to allow immediate and rapid fluid replacement. Crystalloid rather than colloid solutions and artificial plasma expanders would be good in such a situation. Crystalloids can provide short-term expansion of the intravascular space and rapidly distribute to the extra-cellular fluid, which is also depleted in haemorrhagic shock (Baskett 1999). Crystalloids, however, are rapidly lost from the intravascular space. Colloids will persist but occasionally may exacerbate pulmonary oedema by drawing further fluid into the extracellular tissues (Baskett 1999). Crystalloid solutions such as Hartmann's solution and 0.9 per cent saline are the first-line therapy and should be infused as rapidly as possible until the systolic blood pressure is restored or compatible blood is available. When blood loss representing 2000–3000 ml in a woman in late pregnancy occurs, red cell replacement is required. Uncross-matched group O rhesus-negative or red cell concentrates can be used in an emergency.

Informing the hospital anaesthetist and obstetrician in advance of admission may enable the blood transfusion department and obstetric theatres to be on stand-by as appropriate. Later, fluid replacement will be determined by the blood picture and haematologist involvement may be required. It is important to have accurate documentation of fluid input as well as estimated blood loss.

With continued active bleeding, a Caesarean section is the only way to deliver the baby as the placenta is preventing the baby being born vaginally. Also, cervical dilatation occurring in labour will lead to further blood loss, threatening the lives of both mother and fetus. During transfer into hospital, therefore, discuss the prospect of an emergency Caesarean section with the mother, if possible.

Family support is important and it may be necessary to ensure that child care arrangements are made for any other children. Neighbours may be able to help. The police could be contacted to arrange prompt and safe care of the child and can assist in locating any family members nearby.

Placental abruption

Sections of the placenta, if separated prematurely from the uterine wall, will lead to varying degrees of vaginal bleeding. Fox (1978) found evidence of abruption in routinely examined placentas, suggesting that small episodes of placental abruption are more common than diagnosed clinically. Placenta abruption may, in severe cases, lead to at least two-thirds of the placenta becoming detached and 2000 ml of blood or more being lost from the circulation.

Placental abruption is often unprovoked, with no known cause (Konje and Taylor 1999). However, associated risk factors are previous history of placental abruption, increased parity, cigarette smoking, sudden decompression of the uterus such as following membrane rupture in patients with polyhydramnious and multiple pregnancy, external cephalic version, and placental abnormalities especially circumvallate placenta and abdominal trauma (Konje and Taylor 1999). As with placenta praevia, placental abruption carries the risk of maternal mortality and morbidity due to hypovolaemia.

Clinical presentation

Placental abruption can be asymptomatic and only evident when a retroplacental clot is discovered on routine placental inspection post-delivery. Alternatively, depending on the extent of placental separation, signs vary from a small or moderate vaginal bleeding without any haemorrhagic shock or fetal hypoxia to massive haemorrhage and severely compromised mother and fetus.

Bleeding may be:

- Concealed (Figure 2.2(A)). Separation occurs around the centre of the placenta and blood is retained, forming a retroplacental clot (Lindsay 1997a). The blood may be forced into the myometrium, being referred to as a Couvelaire uterus. There will be uterine pain and shock as the uterus becomes increasingly tense, but no visible vaginal blood loss. It may be difficult to differentiate uterine contractions from the abdominal pain caused by the abruption but, in the case of the latter, the pain is sharp, severe and sudden in onset (Green 1989). This type of bleeding occurs in 20–35 per cent of cases (Fraser and Watson 1989).
- Revealed (Figure 2.2(B)). The site of detachment is at the edge of the placenta and blood escapes vaginally (Lindsay 1997a). The visible amount of bleeding correlates with the level of maternal shock observed. Revealed haemorrhage occurs in 65–80 per cent of cases (Fraser and Watson 1989).
- Mixed. There may be a combination of revealed and concealed blood loss. The condition is associated with uterine tenderness and the degree of maternal shock will be out of proportion with the observed vaginal blood loss (Lindsay 1997a).

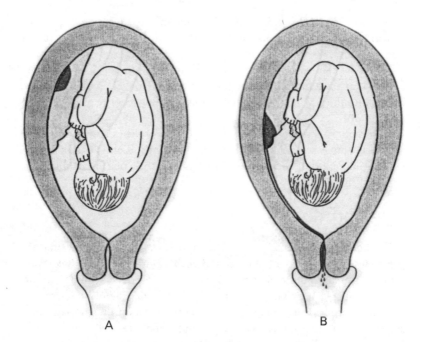

Figure 2.2   A: Concealed abruptio placenta
B: Revealed abruptio placenta

Whether vaginal bleeding is evident or not, if there is marked uterine hardness on palpation, described as feeling 'woody', persistent abdominal pain and maternal shock then a severe placental abruption has occurred. The abdominal girth may increase or a rising fundal height may help in the diagnosis of concealed bleeding (Konje and Taylor 1999).

Concealed bleeding is associated with more severe complications. Shock can occur rapidly in such a situation due to the hypovolaemia, extravasation and consumptive coagulation (tissue damage and the liberation of thromboplastins into the circulation with resulting DIC). Coagulopathy is evident in 30 per cent of cases (Konje and Taylor 1999) and is associated with maternal mortality.

The sign of hypovolaemic shock is predominantly tachycardia, as there is poor correlation between low blood pressure and reduced blood volume in this condition. First, the presence of hypertension may mask true hypovolemia. Secondly, there is a tendency to underestimate blood loss in placental abruption owing to the concealed bleeding into the myometrium.

There is often associated fetal compromise. However, it is important to note that auscultation may be difficult with a Couvelaire uterus (blood forced into the myometrium which infiltrates between the muscle fibres of the uterus).

Feto-maternal haemorrhage can lead to severe rhesus sensitisation in rhesus negative women. Fetal anaemia and transient coagulopathies have been reported in newborns of women with placental abruption (Green 1989).

Management

In community situations, such as the home or a midwifery-led unit, the principles of management of placental abruption with maternal compromise are similar to those discussed under placenta praevia. That is, immediate transfer to hospital via paramedic ambulance should be arranged and monitoring of maternal and fetal condition and fluid replacement should be commenced as soon as possible. The fetal heart may not be heard owing to the Couvelaire uterus, so the midwife should not assume too much when the fetal heart appears undetectable on auscultation. Fluid replacement should be commenced as soon as possible. Because of an association between abruption, pre-eclampsia and DIC (Benedetti 1996), investigative blood tests need to be taken as soon as possible.

The midwife should be alert for signs of labour. Labour may begin spontaneously and progress rapidly. This is due to the irritability of the blood in the uterine muscles. Labour can be advantageous in this situation, as the uterus contracting controls the bleeding. However, postpartum haemorrhage may occur as a result of the Couvelaire uterus, which renders the living ligature action of the muscles less effective following placental separation.

Postpartum haemorrhage

Predisposing factors

There are many factors that increase the risk of a woman having a PPH. During pregnancy these are polyhydramnios, grand multiparity, placenta praevia, previous history of PPH, multiple pregnancies, placental abruption and presence of fibroids. In labour the predisposing factors include prolonged labour, augmented labour, retained placenta or placental products, chorioamnionitis, mismanagement of the third stage and, finally, coagulopathy will increase the risk of haemorrhage. Known risks for coagulopathy include history of abnormal bleeding, a dead fetus, abruption, and HELLP syndrome (haemolysis, elevated liver enzymes and low platelets). However, many cases of primary PPH occur in normal labours with no explanation, and midwives caring for women in labour at home or in a community-based birth centre need to be prepared to manage this emergency.

Clinical presentation of primary PPH

There are four possible causes of PPH, all of which present differently: uterine atony, retained placenta, trauma to the genital tract, and coagulopathy. The ALSO Advanced Life Support in Obstetrics course (American Academy of Family Physicians 2000) use the mnemonic 'The four Ts' (Tone, Tissue, Trauma and Thrombin) as an aide-mémoire.

Midwives need to be acutely aware of the risk of PPH for, whilst visible bleeding is difficult to miss, there remain problems in recognising PPH. These include underestimation of the blood loss, failure to recognise slow but steady bleeding, and failure to recognise occult bleeding, and the clinical signs and symptoms of blood loss may appear late. Initially, the woman will become tachycardic, pale and clammy. By the time her blood pressure falls, severe blood loss will have occurred. Air hunger and altered level of consciousness are late manifestations of PPH.

Immediate assessment, diagnosis of the cause of PPH and management

Uterine atony (Tone)

Uterine atony presents classically as a boggy, soft uterus and accounts for 75 per cent of PPH (American Academy of Family Physicians 2000). Haemorrhage occurs because the living ligature effect of the myometrial muscles fails to occlude the maternal sinuses once the placenta separates.

Massive PPH usually occurs within the first hour after delivery (Bonnar 2000). The management of the third stage of labour has been well researched. There is good quality of evidence that supports the recommendation of active management involving the use of oxytocic drugs in the third stage of labour because of a reduced risk of postpartum haemorrhage (Prendiville and Elbourne 1989). However, Featherstone (1999) found considerable uncertainty among midwives regarding the safe management of the physiological third stage and suggests that further education and experience in conducting the physiological third stage may contribute to a reduced risk of PPH. Nonetheless, PPH may still occur. It is advisable that if a woman states a preference for a physiological third stage during pregnancy the midwife discusses the possibility of administering an oxytocic drug if a PPH should occur. The reason for all procedures necessary to manage postpartum haemorrhage should be explained to the woman and consent obtained before these are undertaken. Management of PPH will be determined by whether or not the placenta has been delivered.

Placenta not delivered (Tissue)
Retained placenta is defined as a failure to deliver the placenta within 30 minutes after birth and occurs in 3 per cent of vaginal deliveries (American Academy of Family Physicians 2000). Whilst ALSO advocate active management, during a physiological third stage of labour the placenta may take up to an hour to be expelled. Local NHS hospitals and birth centres will have policies that define retained placenta, which should guide midwifery practice. The independent midwife may wish to make an assessment based on clinical judgement rather than time. However she would be recommended to liaise with the local supervisor of midwives. Once the diagnosis of retained placenta is made, the woman should be transferred from the home or midwifery-led unit into hospital by paramedic ambulance for treatment. This may involve manual removal of the placenta under regional or general anaesthesia.

Where the placenta remains completely attached to the uterine wall, bleeding from the maternal sinuses will not occur. However, separation may occur at any time and in cases of partial separation, bleeding may be continuous and profuse. Action is urgently required.

MANAGEMENT OF RETAINED PLACENTA
- Call for assistance; do not leave the woman alone.
- 'Rub up' a contraction (Figure 2.3). If the bleeding begins before the placenta is delivered, massage the uterus to 'rub up' a contraction.

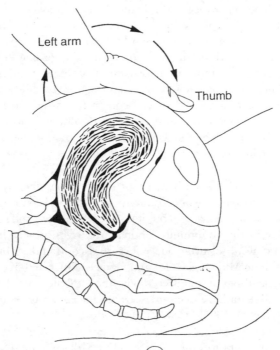

The left hand is cupped over the uterus ( ) and massages it within a firm circular motion in a clockwise direction

Figure 2.3 Rubbing up a contraction

Bleeding is a sign that the placenta is separating or has separated, and only by emptying the uterus of the placenta will the myometrium be able to contract sufficiently to control bleeding for the maternal sinuses.

- Administer an oxytocic drug and attempt to deliver the placenta by controlled cord traction.

The midwife should obtain consent to administer an oxytocic drug if one has not already been given or to give a second dose and attempt to deliver the placenta by CCT. Syntocinon® (oxytocin) 5 units given intramuscularly will normally cause the uterus to contract, therefore aiding placental separation and control of bleeding in two and a half minutes. Syntrometrine® comprising 5 units oxytocin and 0.5 mg ergometrine will act in two and a half minutes if given intramuscularly and 45 seconds if given intravenously. Similarly, ergometrine 0.25–0.5 mg injection acts within the same timeframes according to the route of administration. No more than two doses of either Syntometrine® or ergometrine injection should be administered by midwives because ergometrine causes peripheral vasoconstriction which may result in a sharp rise in blood pressure. However, although for this reason ergometrine is not regarded as first choice for routine use, it produces a prolonged contraction of up to 60 to 90 minutes and is a good second choice.

If available, Hemabate® (carboprost tromethamine) by deep intra-muscular injection will work within five minutes and controls 80 per cent of postpartum haemorrhages but it is kept refrigerated and so has limited availability in the community setting. Midwives are reminded of the need to be aware of drug side effects and contraindications in accor-dance with the Midwives Rules and Code of Practice (UKCC 1998).

Oxytocic drugs administered via the umbilical cord in cases of retained placenta have been investigated but found to be of no benefit (Makkonen et al. 1995, Ozcan et al. 1996).

If no oxytocic drugs are available, unclamp the placental end and allow the placenta to drain, which reduces placental size and thereby aids uterine contraction. Attempt placental delivery by maternal effort in the supine position. It may help to place a hand flat on the lower abdomen above the pubic bone to give the woman something 'to push against' and to press gently upwards whilst applying tension without traction on the cord.

Cord traction should be avoided, as this may lead to risk of cord rupture and uterine inversion when no oxytocic drugs have been admin-istered.

- Empty the bladder and try again to deliver the placenta. If resistance is felt when applying controlled traction to deliver the placenta, catheterise to empty the bladder and try again.
- Monitor the woman for level of shock and administer replacement fluids as described earlier in the chapter.
- If, after all the above measures, the Midwives Rules and Code of Practice (UKCC 1998) state that midwives should be able to perform manual removal of the placenta and manual examination of the uterus as a life-saving measure, in the absence of medical assistance.

Manual removal of the placenta is a traumatic procedure for the woman, resulting in shock, and it is therefore normally undertaken under general/spinal anaesthetic. If not undertaken correctly, the further life-threatening complications of inverted uterus (Stables 1999) uterine rupture and infection may occur (Crafter 2002). The question of whether the midwife in this situation should concentrate on replacing lost fluid and arranging transferring into hospital or attempt manual removal is open to controversy. The midwife should not attempt manual removal unless specific training has been undertaken. The principles of manual removal are described below:

PRINCIPLES FOR MANUAL REMOVAL OF THE PLACENTA
(CRAFTER 2002, LINDSAY 1997B) (FIGURE 2.4)
- A strict aseptic technique should be used.
- The midwife's hand is formed into a cone shape and inserted into the uterus following the umbilical cord whilst the other hand supports the fundus externally, avoiding it being pushed upwards.

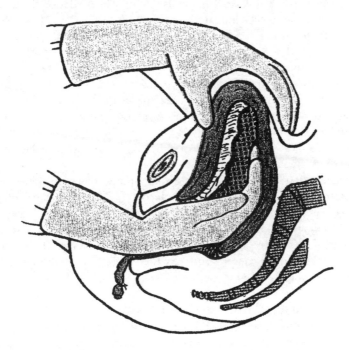

Figure 2.4 Manual removal of the placenta

- The cord is followed to where it inserts into the placenta and the separated area of edge of the placenta is then located. With a gentle 'sawing' movement (Lindsay 1997b p. 709) of the hand between the placenta and the uterine wall, the placenta is separated. Once it is ensured that all placental fragments have been removed from the placental site, the placenta is grasped and removed, taking care to support the uterus to prevent uterine inversion.
- Following the manual removal, Syntometrine® or ergometrine should be administered to achieve a strong uterine contraction, and the woman should be urgently transferred to hospital by paramedic ambulance.

Placenta delivered

MANAGEMENT

- If the bleeding begins after delivery of the placenta, call for assistance.
- Uterine massage will expel any clots that may be hindering the uterus to contract and will stimulate a contraction.
- Administer an oxytocic drug. If appropriate, encourage the mother to breastfeed as this will stimulate uterine contraction.
- Ensure that the bladder is empty.
- You may want to raise the woman's feet to delay her feeling faint from the blood loss, but do not raise the foot of the bed, as this may cause pooling of blood in the uterus, inhibiting effective contraction (Stables 1999).
- Monitor the woman for level of shock and administer replacement fluids as soon as possible.
- Examination of the placenta and membranes for completeness will establish whether or not retained placental tissue is the cause of the bleeding.
- If bleeding continues following the administration of oxytocic drugs, bimanual compression may be performed externally. If this fails, internal bimanual compression may be required to control the bleeding from the placental site.

EXTERNAL BIMANUAL COMPRESSION
External bimanual compression is where one hand follows the curve of the uterus abdominally in order to get as posterior as possible, while the other hand is placed on the flat of the abdomen. Pressure is applied by

compressing the two hands together and upwards. This applies pressure to the bleeding placental bed and straightens the uterine veins, relieving congestion and decreasing the bleeding (Lindsay 1997b).

INTERNAL BIMANUAL COMPRESSION (FIGURE 2.5)
Internal bimanual compression is more readily described in the literature but it may cause shock if conducted without adequate anaesthesia. It should therefore only be undertaken where other measures have failed to control haemorrhage.

One hand is inserted into the vagina forced into a fist and pushed in an upwards direction towards the anterior vaginal fornix (Lindsay

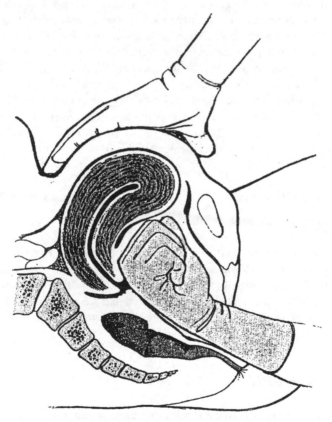

Figure 2.5   Internal bimanual compression

1997b). The other, external hand dips down behind the fundus and pulls it forwards towards the symphysis pubis in order to compress the placental site. The procedure is maintained until the uterus remains contracted.

The midwife should accompany the woman during transfer to hospital by paramedic ambulance undertaken as soon as possible.

Haemorrhage due to trauma

Trauma to the genital tract can also be a cause of postpartum haemorrhage. Trauma can include lacerations and haematomas and, less commonly, uterine inversion and uterine rupture (these latter two causes are beyond the scope of this chapter). In cases of cervical, vaginal wall, clitoral, labial and perineal lacerations, diagnosis is made when bleeding is observed despite the uterus being well contracted. Cervical tears can be difficult to suture in a home birth situation owing to inadequate exposure and friable oedematous tissue. Applying ring forceps to the bleeding edges and leaving them in place for several hours may be necessary. A high vaginal wall tear with an intact perineum can cause a continuous trickle of blood. The midwife should always inspect carefully for genital tract trauma following a birth so that there is no delay in recognising the potential severity of this situation. Direct pressure or artery forceps to bleeding vessels should be applied and the trauma sutured as soon as possible. If bleeding continues despite the suturing of visible trauma, transfer to hospital for further investigation and treatment should be arranged.

Coagulopathy (Thrombin)

Coagulopathy is the least common cause of PPH but a frequent consequence. Its clinical presentation is the blood not forming clots and the woman not responding to the usual treatment for PPH. Urgent transfer into a consultant obstetric unit by paramedic ambulance is required. Accurate documentation of blood loss estimation and replacement of blood loss is essential. Dextran infusion should be avoided as it can prolong bleeding time and may interfere with cross-matching when the woman is hospitalised.

Secondary PPH

Secondary PPH is usually the result of retained products of conception. Other causes include the presence of a blood clot, fibroid or intrauterine infection. Heavy red, offensive lochia and a very tender, subinvoluted uterus are also indications. Infection can also give rise to a low-grade pyrexia and tachycardia. If haemorrhage occurs, commonly 7 to 14 days after delivery (Lindsay 1997b), the management is similar as for primary PPH with a delivered placenta, with measures taken to stop the bleeding by rubbing up a contraction, administration of an oxytocic drug, emptying the bladder and commencing fluid replacement. The mother and baby should be transferred to the obstetric consultant unit by paramedic ambulance.

Conclusion

Major obstetric haemorrhage occurring in the community setting will undoubtedly present the midwife with a challenge. It is important that all members of the multidisciplinary team are utilised for the expertise they can provide. Paramedics will provide essential support and skills to the midwife in the home setting and outlying midwifery-led units – for example canulation and infusion expertise – until such time as the woman can be transported into hospital for medical assessment and management. This chapter has provided a framework for the immediate assessment and management of major obstetric haemorrhage in the community.

Supervisor of midwives' commentary

The chapter has highlighted some of the difficulties in defining massive obstetric haemorrhage in that it is often defined after the event. This chapter is very easy to read and is worth reviewing on a regular basis.

Antepartum haemorrhage

Occasionally the difficulty with women who have placenta praevia is that they most definitely do not want to stay in hospital from 36 weeks' gestation. I am sure we have all been aware of situations where women sit in an antenatal ward from Monday to Friday and then go home for weekend leave. As if bleeding is less likely to happen during the weekend! If the risk has been assessed as great enough for a woman to be admitted to hospital for the week, this risk does not change at the weekend. Women should be encouraged to stay, with reasons for this decision explained. Details of the situation and the information given should of course be recorded in the women's notes.

As midwives, we are only too aware of the potential for disaster with these women. But the woman, who feels perfectly well, will almost certainly not have the background knowledge or experience to know that bleeding can be unheralded, torrential and catastrophic for her and her baby.

Midwives are reminded that their supervisor of midwives will be available to offer them clinical advice and support in dealing with such a difficult situation.

As a supervisor of midwives, I was recently made aware of a concealed placental abruption. The woman presented with some abdominal pain, she had no recognisable risk factors and her clinical observations did not cause any concern. Within an hour of her initial assessment her condition had deteriorated so rapidly that an emergency Caesarean section was necessary. Whilst we are not likely to be presented with such a situation on a regular basis, we are likely to find ourselves offering advice to women regarding abdominal pain. It is essential, therefore, that we remain vigilant and receptive at all times to the information we give and are given. The midwife involved in this situation certainly was and, as a result, the outcome was good.

Postpartum haemorrhage

The midwife's action and her plan for management will depend on the findings of her immediate assessment. Use of the four Ts, presented within the chapter, provides a guideline as to what must be considered as causes of the bleeding.

In relation to the administration of an oxytocic drug, consideration must be made here as to whether the woman has previously indicated that she does not wish to have an oxytocic drug administered. The chapter reminds us that we must keep the woman informed of the situation; she may recognize the urgency for intervention and consent to the administration of oxytocic drugs. If this is not the case and a midwife is managing a primary PPH in the community setting, we are reminded of the fundamental principles of managing such a case.

Undoubtedly this will be a traumatic experience for all concerned and seeking clinical or statutory supervision after such an event is, therefore, strongly recommended, as is ensuring regular updating on managing a PPH in the safe environment of a classroom during skills and drills updates.

Key points

- Access medical aid as soon as possible. Call for assistance – paramedics will be extremely useful in this type of situation.

- In cases of PPH, stem the flow of bleeding.
- Monitor the condition of the woman and fetus.
- Implement fluid replacement as a matter of urgency.
- Ensure contemporaneous record-keeping of proceedings.

Anaesthetist's commentary

Obstetric haemorrhage can be a life-threatening event, a rate of 3.3 deaths per million maternities was quoted in the most recent triennial Confidential Enquiries into Maternal Deaths. In addition, a recent survey (Waterstone et al. 2001) of severe maternal morbidity suggests that severe, possibly life-threatening, haemorrhage may occur in 6.7 per 1000 deliveries, which means that there could be around fourteen hundred cases of severe haemorrhage in the UK every year.

The following case description from the triennial Confidential Enquiries into Maternal Deaths (NICE 2001 p. 98) reinforces how devastating obstetric haemorrhage can be.

A multiparous woman with a number of previous caesarean sections (the first for strong fetal indications, the following elective) was diagnosed as having placenta praevia on ultrasound scan at about 20 weeks of gestation. She had recurrent episodes of bleeding from then on and was managed as an inpatient from 25 weeks of gestation onwards. The risk of placenta accreta and major haemorrhage was repeatedly discussed with the woman and among all relevant staff, and detailed multidisciplinary plans were made for a planned caesarean section at 36 weeks and for an emergency section should bleeding or labour occur before this. Heavy bleeding, in the early hours of the morning, did occur just before the planned section and the prepared plan was immediately put into action. Surgery, including caesarean section, a hysterectomy and cross-clamping of the aorta was performed by three consultant obstetricians and a consultant vascular surgeon. The consultant anaesthetist was fully supported by staff from the intensive care unit (ICU) and extra experienced midwifery and theatre staff were on duty. Sixty units of blood were given in the first two hours and 200 units in all. After a few hours the situation appeared to be temporarily stable and she was transferred to ICU. Unfortunately, further bleeding occurred and she eventually died a few weeks later without recovering consciousness.

This demonstrates how difficult management can be, even in a hospital setting with excellent preparation.

The preceding chapter gives an excellent description of causes and management of obstetric haemorrhage. Drawing on the recommendations of the CEMD about haemorrhage, a few points must be further emphasised.

The speed with which obstetric haemorrhage can become life-threatening emphasises the need for women at known high risk of haemorrhage to be delivered in a hospital with a blood bank on site and appropriate laboratory facilities, including haematological advice and therapy. However, the unexpected will happen, and relating to emergencies in the community preparation is essential. Every delivery unit should have a protocol for management of obstetric haemorrhage. It is strongly recommended to obtain a copy of your local unit's protocol and carry it – it is extremely useful to have a checklist to hand in emergencies.

One of the most important points to stress is that it is difficult to assess blood loss. People generally underestimate, and blood pressure is a poor indicator of the amount of bleeding. In the young, the sympathetic nervous system can often maintain systolic blood pressure until 30 per cent of total blood volume has been lost (up to 1500 ml). By the time blood pressure is falling, the woman is in severe shock and recovery may be difficult. Tachycardia is often an early sign, although the stress of labour and delivery may cause some confusion. It is important to obtain intravenous access early and commence fluid resuscitation. My personal opinion, mirrored by the Advanced Trauma Life Support for Doctors course (American College of Surgeons 1997) is that, as a minimum, a 16-gauge cannula must be sited early if there is any concern.

Which fluid to use continues to be a matter of debate (colloid v crystalloid) (Hinds and Watson, 1996, p. 86). However, if a patient is bleeding, what is more important is to start giving fluid as quickly as possible. In the acute phase there is no evidence that one fluid is better than another, please be guided by local protocols.

In managing haemorrhage in the hospital, it is important that experienced consultant obstetric and anaesthetic staff attend and that haematological advice and therapy be immediately available. Relating to the community setting, it is essential to arrange transfer to hospital as quickly as possible. In addition, an emergency ambulance gives the additional resources of skilled paramedics, oxygen and additional intravenous fluids. Warning the delivery unit is essential – this allows valuable time to mobilise senior staff, prepare theatre and warn haematology that blood may be required rapidly.

Problem-based scenario and interactive action planning exercise
An emergency primary postpartum haemorrhage following
planned home birth

Anna has just given birth to a large, healthy baby at home, as planned. You notice a large gush of blood with the delivery of the baby. Anna has requested a physiological third stage.

Make your clinical assessment
What factors in your assessment of Anna is helping you make an initial diagnosis?

Care planning
What would your initial plan of care be?

Your answer should include the following:

- Palpate the uterus to assess tone.
- Large babies tend to have large placentas and consequently a large placental site. However, large babies are often associated with maternal anaemia and the threshold of blood loss should be reduced accordingly. Close observation of the blood loss is essential.
- Consider the timing of when Anna last passed urine. Might she have a full bladder inhibiting optimum uterine contraction?
- You may wish to prepare oxytocic drugs and get a catheter ready in case you decide you need to use either.
- Further assistance is important in case the situation deteriorates. DO NOT leave the woman, and continue to observe the lochia without interfering with Anna's first moments with her baby.
- Supporting the baby to breastfeed would be nice in this situation, if appropriate.

The bleeding does not subside, and the umbilical cord is still attached but not pulsating.

What factors in your assessment of Anna will help you decide whether to intervene and suggest an active third stage?

Assessment

- Continue to assess uterine contraction and lochia.
- Blood pressure and pulse can give further clinical features or a base-line for subsequent monitoring.
- Discussion about your concerns with Anna and any family present is important. It is because of your skill and judgement that you are attending Anna for her birth and your communication with her needs to be clear and frequent.
- Consent for oxytocic drugs needs to be gained and maintaining a trusting relationship is important in this situation.
- Remember that PPH can be unpredictable so be prepared and early recognition and prompt treatment is necessary. Inspect the genital tract for trauma which might coexist with uterine atony. It may be that Anna has sustained vaginal injury and that direct pressure and suturing may be required.

Anna can see for herself that the bleeding is heavy and agrees to the administration of oxytocic drugs. The placenta delivers easily following an active management of the third stage. However, Anna continues to bleed more than you would expect. There was no obvious trauma that would explain the blood loss, and the uterus is boggy on palpation.

What would your plan of care be?

You should have identified the following points:

- Request paramedic ambulance assistance and transfer to hospital, and further midwifery/GP support.
- Explain the need for all active intervention to Anna. In an emergency you still require consent if possible.
- Rub up a contraction and expel any blood clots.
- Catheterise the bladder in case a full bladder is hindering contraction and retraction of the uterine muscles.
- Administer Syntometrine® or ergometrine.
- Inspect the placenta for completeness.
- Insert IV cannula if you have undertaken the appropriate training (paramedics will assist).

→

→

- Evaluate Anna's condition while awaiting further assistance: pulse, respiration, colour and blood pressure, whether or not the uterus is well contracted, and the amount of bleeding.
- You may want to raise her feet to delay her feeling faint from the blood loss.
- Discuss the transfer into hospital with the family. The mother would not want to be separated from her baby and so the baby needs to be cared for following its birth and dressed warmly for the journey.
- Encouraging Anna to breastfeed will help the uterus to contract.
- Estimate how much blood she is losing. If the bleeding remains profuse and you are concerned that her condition is deteriorating, commence external bimanual compression.
- If this is unsuccessful in controlling the bleeding, undertake internal bimanual compression.
- Document, even if in rough, the time at which you carry out the care that you do so that you are able to make an accurate record in full at a later stage.
- Cannulate with two 14-gauge cannulae before peripheral shutdown occurs. Administer crystalloid and artificial plasma expanders.
- Continue on-going monitoring – frequently assess uterine contraction and observe lochia. An indwelling catheter, if available, will enable hourly output to assist in evaluating Anna's condition.
- Keep accurate documentation of estimated blood loss and fluid input.
- Accompany Anna to hospital in order to provide care en route if necessary. Inform labour ward and ask them to inform the full obstetric emergency team/discuss the situation with the registrar or consultant on call.

References

American Academy of Family Physicians (2000) *ALSO Provider Course Syllabus* (4th edn). ALSO: Leawood, KS.

American College of Surgeons (1997) *Advanced Trauma Life Support for Doctors*. American College of Surgeons: Chicago.

Baskett T F (1999) *Essential Management of Obstetric Emergencies* (3rd edn). Clinical Press Ltd: Bristol.

Benedetti T J (1996) Obstetric Hemorrhage. In S G Gabble, J R Niebyl, J L Simpson (eds) *Obstetrics: Normal and Problem Pregnancies* (3rd edn) Churchill Livingstone: London.

Bonnar J (2000) Massive Obstetric Haemorrhage, *Baillière's Clinical Obstetrics and Gynaecology* **14** (1), 1–18.

Crafter H (2002) Intrapartum and Primary Postpartum Haemorrhage in Boyle M (ed) *Emergencies Around Childbirth* Radcliffe Medical Press: Oxford.

Featherstone I E (1999) Physiological third stage of labour, *British Journal of Midwifery* **7** (4), 216–21.

Fox H (1978) *Pathology of the Placenta*, W B Saunders: London.

Fraser R and Watson R (1989) Bleeding During the Latter Half of Pregnancy. In I Chalmers (ed), *Effective Care in Pregnancy and Childbirth* Oxford University Press: Oxford.

Green J R (1989) Placenta Abnormalities: Placenta Praevia and Abruptio Placentae. In R K Creasy and R Resnik (eds), *Maternal-Fetal Medicine: Principles and Practice*. W B Saunders: Philadelphia; PA.

Hibbard B M (1988) Bleeding in Late Pregnancy. In B M Hibbard (ed.), *Principles of Obstetrics* Butterworths: London.

Hinds C and Watson D (1996) *Intensive Care: A Concise Textbook* W B Saunders: London.

Konje J C and Taylor D J (1999) Bleeding in Late Pregnancy. In D K James, P J Steer, C P Weiner, B Gonik (eds), *High Risk Pregnancy – Management Options* (2nd edn) W B Saunders: London.

Lindsay P (1997a) Bleeding in Pregnancy in B R Sweet with D Tiran (eds), *Mayes' Midwifery. A Textbook for Midwives* (12th edn). London: Baillière Tindall.

Lindsay P (1997b) Complications of the Third Stage of Labour in B R Sweet with D Tiran (eds), *Mayes' Midwifery. A Textbook for Midwives* (12th edn). London: Baillière Tindall.

Makkonen M, Suonio S and Saarikkoski S (1995) Intraumbilical Oxytocin for Management of Retained Placenta, *International Journal of Gynecology and Obstetrics* **48**, 169–72.

McClelland DBL (ed) (1995) *Optimal Use of Donor Blood. Report from a Working Party set up by the Clinical Resource and Audit Group*. The Scottish Office: Edinburgh.

NICE (National Institute for Clinical Excellence) (2001) *Why Mothers Die 1997–1999; The Confidential Enquiries into Maternal Deaths in the United Kingdom* Royal College Obstetricians and Gynaecology Press: London.

NICE (National Institute for Clinical Excellence) (2003) *Antenatal Care: Routine Care for the Healthy Pregnant Woman*. NICE: London.

Ozcan T, Sahin G and Senoz S (1996) The Effect of Intraumbilical Oxytocin on the Third Stage of Labour, *Australian and New Zealand Journal of Obstetrics and Gynaecology* **36**, 9–11.

Prendiville W and Elbourne D (1989) Care During the Third Stage of Labor. In L Chalmers, M Enkin, M J N C Keirse (eds), *Effective Care in Pregnancy and Childbirth*, Vol. 2, 1145–70. Oxford University Press: Oxford.

Sakhry S M and Sheldon G F (1994) Massive Transfusion in the Surgical Patient. In LC Jefferies and M E Brecher (eds), *Massive Transfusion*. American Association of Blood Banks: Bethesda; MD.

Scott (1986) Antepartum Haemorrhage. In C R Whitfield (ed), *Dewhurst's Textbook of Obstetrics and Gynaecology for Postgraduates* (4th edn). Blackwell Scientific Publications: Oxford.

Stables D (1999) *Physiology in Childbearing with Anatomy and Related Biosciences*. Baillière Tindall: London.

Sweet B R with Tiran D (eds) (1997) *Mayes' Midwifery. A Textbook for Midwives* (12th edn). Baillière Tindall: London.

UKCC (United Kingdom Central Council for Nursing, Midwifery and Health Visiting) (1998) *Midwives Rules and Code of Practice*. UKCC: London.

Waterstone M, Bewley S and Wolfe C (2001) Incidence and Predictors of Severe Obstetric Morbidity: Case Control Study, *British Medical Journal* **322**, 1089–93.

3

Pre-eclampsia and the Emergency Management of Eclampsia outside the Hospital

Nicki Young

Introduction

Pre-eclampsia is the most common complication of pregnancy, affecting one in ten pregnancies overall in the United Kingdom (Action on Pre-eclampsia 2000). In the majority of cases, symptoms will be mild and the pregnancy will result in a healthy baby. However one in every fifty women will suffer severe illness and the outcome will be poor. It is this group of women who are at highest risk of developing one of the crises associated with pre-eclampsia, the most well known being eclampsia. According to Douglas and Redman (1994), eclampsia complicates nearly one in two thousand pregnancies. The most recent Confidential Enquiry into Maternal Deaths (CEMD) in the United Kingdom (NICE 2001) records 15 deaths due to pre-eclampsia or eclampsia. The condition also contributes to the perinatal mortality rate, being responsible for the deaths of between five and six hundred babies each year (Action on Pre-eclampsia 2000). Each death is a tragedy for the parents and family involved. The condition can also bring considerable physical and psychological morbidity to the survivors.

Although the mortality rate associated with pre-eclampsia reported in the latest CEMD (NICE 2001) represents a reduction from previous reports, substandard care continues to be highlighted. Examples were given of primary health care professionals failing to appreciate the significance of symptoms, failing to understand the significance of past obstetric history and planning care accordingly, and performing inadequate assessments. Salha and Walker (1999) believe that the answer to substandard care and poor management of eclampsia lies partly in better education and training of all health care professionals.

During the literature search and review for this chapter, very little was found on the management of eclampsia outside the hospital environment. Although eclampsia is uncommon in the UK today, it remains a life-threatening event. The British Eclampsia Survey (Douglas and Redman 1994) found that a quarter of all eclamptic fits occurred outside the hospital, and therefore health professionals need to be prepared to manage this obstetric emergency wherever it occurs. However, primary care health workers face a different set of problems from their counterparts in the hospital environment, as many work either alone or in an environment with limited resources and personnel. Consequently, it is imperative that they keep up to date with contemporary knowledge and treatment of the condition and have prepared action plans to manage the emergency.

Owing to the apparent gap in the literature relating to care of the eclamptic woman in the community, the overall aim of this chapter is to explore the principles of management and care during an eclamptic fit that occurs outside the hospital environment. However, to understand why a woman's condition has deteriorated into a crisis, the condition of pre-eclampsia needs to be studied. The chapter is, therefore, divided into two parts. The first will explore the following areas:

- the underlying pathophysiology and how this relates to the myriad of signs and symptoms;
- progression of the pre-eclampsia process;
- eclampsia;
- the principles of management and care of an eclamptic fit when it occurs outside the hospital environment.

Surveillance during the child-bearing continuum

According to Marsh and Renfrew (1999), community midwives are the lead carers in over 80 per cent of pregnancies and specialists are involved only by referral. The chapter in the latest CEMD (NICE 2001) focusing on midwifery practice highlights the crucial role the midwife plays in antenatal, intrapartum and postnatal surveillance. Surveillance includes assessing maternal and fetal risk factors and screening to detect the signs and symptoms of pre-eclampsia. Once an abnormality is detected, the midwife will refer the woman to the appropriate medical practitioner for further investigations and monitoring. Working within local trust guidelines, the midwife will judge the appropriate intervals to allow between screening assessments.

However, the midwife must bear in mind that pre-eclampsia can occur at any stage in the pregnancy and often in the early stages of the condition the woman may be symptomless. As the condition progresses, symptoms will inevitably become apparent. According to Redman (2002 p. 181) the condition is unpredictable and can evolve over a short period of time, 'often within two weeks'. When eclampsia occurs in gestations before 37 weeks it appears to have more severe complications for the mother and baby. Preterm birth has consequences for the baby, as immaturity and the effects of the pre-eclampsia process may lead to perinatal mortality or morbidity (Douglas and Redman 1994, Mattar and Sibai 2000). Regular antenatal care is, therefore, vitally important to screen for asymptomatic and early onset pre-eclampsia (Redman 2002). However, it must be acknowledged that there may be a downside to rigorous screening. Some women will be referred, and undergo tests and investigations, even though they may not go on to develop the condition, this may result in increased levels of stress and anxiety. Guidance on the frequency of antenatal appointments and screening for pre-eclampsia can be found in the clinical guideline relating to antenatal care for the healthy pregnant woman (NCCWCH 2003). Although this document was commissioned by the National Institute for Clinical Excellence (NICE) it is a guideline and the midwife retains her responsibility to make an individual assessment of each woman and schedule appointments accordingly (Sidebotham 2004).

Risk factors for pre-eclampsia

To be able to implement a risk management strategy, midwives need to have knowledge of the risk factors associated with the development of pre-eclampsia. Evidence from epidemiological studies has identified a number of factors which can be used in identifying women at risk of the

First pregnancy
Family history of pre-eclampsia-genetic component
Previous history of pre-eclampsia
Body mass index at or above 35 at first contact
Multiple pregnancy
Hydatidiform mole
Renal disease
Chronic hypertension
Diabetes mellitus
Collegan vascular diseases
Rhesus isoimmunisation
Extremes of age; under 20 or over 35 years
Paternity change (protective role of previous antigen
      exposure)

Figure 3.1   Risk factors for pre-eclampsia

disorder (Dekker and Sibai 2001). However, it does not follow that if a woman is free of these factors she will be at no risk of developing the condition. Figure 3.1 lists the risk factors for pre-eclampsia.

Pathophysiology of pre-eclampsia

Pre-eclampsia is a pregnancy-specific progressive disorder triggered by abnormal placentation which leads to vascular endothelial damage. This widespread damage causes a maternal systemic reaction where each end organ may be affected to different degrees, and the effects may be seen in both mother and baby (Nelson-Piercy 2002, Redman and Roberts 1993).

Placental ischaemia

During placental development the spiral arteries need to undergo structural modifications to enable them to deliver the increased blood supply to the placental site. This modification is achieved by an increase in the lumen of the spiral arteries, with the walls being remodelled so they contain very little smooth muscle (Brosens et al. 1967, Roberts and

Cooper 2001). Remodelling occurs as a result of invasion of fetal trophoblast into the maternal vessels, which induces a physiological dilatation of spiral arteries (Roberts and Cooper 2001). These modifications are usually completed by weeks 20–22 (Roberts and Lain 2002). However, they do not occur or only partially occur in the pregnancy complicated with pre-eclampsia, leaving the spiral arteries to retain their endothelial and muscular linings (Khong et al. 1986, Roberts and Cooper 2001).

This reduction in the spiral arteries' capacity to carry an adequate blood supply to the placenta results in a reduction in intervillous blood flow and leads to impaired placental function (Duckett et al. 2001). Consequently, placental ischaemia and hypoxia ensues, which leads to fetal intrauterine growth restriction. The inability of the trophoblast to penetrate and widen the spiral arteries of the uterus appears to have a genetic and immunological basis (Roberts and Cooper 2001, Duckett et al. 2001).

Endothelial cell damage

The underperfusion of the placenta and ischaemia leads to the production of an as yet unidentified factor, which is released into the maternal circulation (Myers and Baker 2002, Roberts et al. 1989). This factor appears to target the endothelial cells lining organs and vessels causing damage leading to an alteration in their function and resulting in the maternal syndrome. The site and extent of endothelial cell damage will dictate the initial signs and symptoms of the syndrome (Duckett et al. 2001, Myers and Baker 2002). The following is an outline of some of the features of endothelial cell damage (Duckett et al. 2001, Roberts et al. 1989, Roberts and Redman 1993):

- increase in vascular sensitivity to pressor agents (i.e. angiotensin II) leading to vasoconstriction;
- the balance between thromboxane (vasoconstrictor) and prostacyclin (vasodilator) synthesis shifts towards thromboxane leading to vasospasm and vasoconstriction of blood vessels;
- vasospasm leading to ischaemia;
- vasoconstriction leading to increased blood pressure;
- reduced blood volume and haemoconcentration;
- reduction in organ perfusion;

- loss of endothelial integrity which leads to fluid loss from intravascular compartments into tissues leading to oedema;
- glomerular endothelial cells become increasingly permeable resulting in proteinuria;
- hypoalbuminaemia causes a lower colloid pressure altering fluid transport across capillaries;
- decreased endothelial production of prostacyclin (platelet inhibitor);
- reduced production of prostacyclin increasing the thromboxane/prostacyclin ratio (prostacyclin inhibits platelet agregation; thromboxane promotes it);
- endothelial cell damage causes platelet activation leading to thrombocytopenia.

Signs and symptoms

The development of pre-eclampsia is often characterised as the dyad of new hypertension arising after the twentieth week of pregnancy in association with proteinuria. Many sources take the classification system accepted by the International Society for the Study of Hypertension in Pregnancy (ISSHP) (Davey and MacGillivray 1988). The following definition of hypertension has been adapted from Churchill and Beevers (1999), which reflects the ISSHP system.

Hypertension defined as either:

- one measurement of diastolic blood pressure of more than 110 mmHg or
- two consecutive measurements of diastolic blood pressure of 90 mmHg or more at least 4 hours apart or
- threshold rises in the systolic and diastolic levels.

The absolute value of the blood pressure is not the only important factor; a rise in blood pressure above the earliest recorded pregnancy reading also needs to be considered.

This includes a rise in the systolic blood pressure of 30 mmHg or more and diastolic blood pressure of 15 mmHg or more when compared with the first trimester blood pressure, on two consecutive occasions four or more hours apart (Churchill and Beevers 1999 p. 5).

The following definition of proteinuria has been taken from the antenatal care clinical guideline (NCCWCH 2003 p. 101). Consideration must be given to the fact that dipstick testing for protein is very inaccurate (Nelson-Piercy 2002).

Significant proteinuria defined as:

- 1 + proteinuria or greater on dipstick. This needs to be confirmed by a twenty-four hour urinary measurement;
- a total protein excretion of 300 mg or more in a twenty-four hour urine collection.

It is essential to remember that, as a feature of pre-eclampsia, an increase in blood pressure may occur as an early or late feature or may be mild (Churchill and Beevers 1999). Although hypertension and proteinuria are the most common manifestations of pre-eclampsia there is 'enormous variation in the severity, timing, progression and order of onset of different clinical features' (Nelson-Piercy 2002 p. 7). For example, hypertension does not have to be present or severe, and proteinuria may appear before hypertension. Because pre-eclampsia is a syndrome which can affect any system in the mother and baby, there are a myriad of signs and symptoms that can be exhibited. The woman's individual systemic reaction will dictate the signs and symptoms she exhibits (Walker 2000 p. 1260). Nelson-Piercy (2002 p. 11) explains that in practice the diagnosis of pre-eclampsia 'is made when there is a constellation of recognised features'.

The following are clinical features that can be directly attributable to the pathophysiology of pre-eclampsia and suggest significant end organ involvement. Many of these features are signs of worsening condition and, depending on the woman's overall clinical assessment, she may need immediate referral for investigation and further monitoring.

- severe headache/visual disturbances/photophobia/nausea and vomiting/behaviour changes/irritability/drowsiness/incoherent speech/convulsions
- placental abruption
- rupture/irritation/swelling of the liver capsule due to hypertension causing epigastric pain/liver tenderness/jaundice/nausea and vomiting/Haemolysis, Elevated Liver Enzymes and Low Platelets (HELLP) Syndrome
- proteinuria
- rapidly increasing oedema.

Because pre-eclampsia is a condition of pregnancy it will invariably affect the baby. The effects arise from the nutritional and respiratory deprivation which occurs as a result of placental insufficiency. The effects may be expressed in the following features:

- intrauterine growth restriction
- decreased fetal movements

Laboratory tests are performed to assess pre-eclampsia, and often serial measurements are taken to detect any deterioration. The following tests are taken from McKay (2000).

Abnormal haematological tests:

- reduced plasma volume leading to haemoconcentration may be reflected in an increased haemoglobin level
- decreased platelet count.

Abnormal liver function tests:

- raised aspartate aminotransaminase (AST)
- raised alanine aminotransaminase (ALT)
- raised alkaline phosphatase

(Altered liver function tests may be indicative of HELLP Syndrome).
Abnormal renal function tests:

- Creatinine clearance values (usually assessed via a 24-hour urine collection) may be reduced as a consequence of a fall in glomerular filtration rate
- raised serum creatinine
- raised serum uric acid levels (sensitive marker of disease progression)
- raised urea levels.

Progression of pre-eclampsia

Once pre-eclampsia is established, it will become progressively worse until either the woman is delivered or the condition of the mother or baby deteriorates into a crisis. Figure 3.2 lists the possible crises that may occur as a result of the pre-eclampsia process.

Eclampsia
Cerebral haemorrhage
HELLP syndrome
Hepatic rupture/infarction
Placental abruption
Disseminated intravascular coagulation (DIC)
Renal impairment
Pulmonary oedema/adult respiratory distress syndrome
  (ARDS)
Intrauterine growth restriction
Intrauterine fetal death
Perinatal death

Figure 3.2   Possible crises that may occur as a result of the
pre-eclampsia process

The scenario of an eclamptic fit, included at the end of this chapter, illustrates a linear view of the condition. It follows a classical sequence of hypertension and proteinuria preceding worsening signs and symptoms. However, both Katz et al. (2000) and Douglas and Redman (1994) explain that, because the condition is so unpredictable, we need to move away from the hierarchical view of clinical features. Eclampsia has not been found to be necessarily related to either the degree of proteinuria or the degree of hypertension, and atypical cases will present. It is important to appreciate the enormous variation in how a woman may present with the condition.

Severe or fulminating pre-eclampsia

Fulminating pre-eclampsia is characterised by a sudden decline in the woman's condition due to the severity of signs and symptoms. The condition will become much worse with possibly severe uncontrollable hypertension, and deterioration in the haematological and biochemical investigations (Greer 2001). This period of severity is variable in length and during it the woman is at great risk of suffering one of the crises such as eclampsia or HELLP syndrome (Greer 2001). Macdonald (in Boyle 2002 p. 46) describes fulminating pre-eclampsia as a medical emergency in itself and views it as being the 'window of opportunity' in which intervention and treatment can be actioned in an attempt to prevent a crisis occurring. However, owing to the nature of the pre-eclampsia process not all women will exhibit the signs and symptoms of severe disturbance prior to a crisis occurring. Although convulsions are hazardous and remain a significant cause of maternal mortality, seizures themselves are not often the cause of death; rather it is the 'severity caused by the underlying pathological disturbances' (Douglas and Redman 1994 p. 1399).

Eclampsia

Eclampsia is defined as fitting, associated with pre-eclampsia, which cannot be attributed to other cerebral causes. In the vast majority of cases, eclampsia is preceded by several days or weeks of clinically evident pre-eclampsia, although some cases occur without any premonitory signs or symptoms (Kean et al. 2000).

The Eclampsia Survey (Douglas and Redman 1994), conducted throughout the UK in 1992, recorded 383 confirmed cases of eclampsia. These cases were analysed in relation to when convulsions occurred. Forty-four per cent of women experienced their first fit in the postnatal period. Thirty-eight per cent experienced eclampsia in the antenatal period and 18 per cent in the intrapartum period.

The survey also showed a maternal mortality of 1 in 50 and a peri-natal mortality rate of 1 in 14. In the week before the first convulsion 325 women had been seen by a doctor or midwife. The features documented at the antenatal visit preceding the eclamptic fit are listed in Table 3.1. (adapted from Douglas and Redman 1994).

Table 3.1   Presence of hypertension or proteinuria

Presence of hypertension or proteinuria	Number (%) (n = 325)
Neither proteinuria nor hypertension	36 (11)
Proteinuria alone	32 (10)
Hypertension alone	71 (22)
Both proteinuria and hypertension	186 (57)

Pathophysiology of eclampsia

Although the pathophysiology of eclampsia is not completely established, a number of explanations are proposed (Duckett et al. 2001). Cerebral vasospasm and vasoconstriction may result in reduced perfusion which leads to cerebral ischaemia, disrupting the blood brain barrier and leading to cerebral oedema (Barton et al. 1992, Salha and Walker 1999). This may cause abnormal electrical activity leading to a convulsion. The vasoconstriction and intensity of the blood pressure may rupture blood vessels leading to cerebral haemorrhage. According to Redman and Roberts (1993 p. 1453) 'eclamptic seizures vary from mild self-limited events' to cases of 'profound intracerebral pathology'. Although the majority of women convulse once, there may be considerable morbidity (Walker 1996).

Eclampsia may be signalled by the classic signs of headache, visual disturbances and epigastric pain (Greer in Chamberlain and Steer 2001). Sibai (1990) found blurred vision, photophobia, irritability, transient mental changes and nausea and vomiting were also signs warning of an imminent fit.

Stages of a fit

There are defined stages during an eclamptic fit as described in Table 3.2 (adapted from ALSO 1996, MacKeigan 2000 and Usta and Sibai 1995). During the fit the mother is at risk of aspiration of vomit or blood and she may injure herself. A severe rise in blood pressure may lead to increased intracranial pressure and predispose to cerebral vascular accident and recurrent convulsions. Most eclamptic fits resolve in 60 to 90 seconds (Witlin 1999). Although about 35 per cent of women will reconvulse, they probably do so about half an hour to an hour later (Walker 2003).

Perinatal outcome

If the fit occurs in the antenatal or intrapartum period it has consequences for the baby. Due to the severe vasospasm of uterine arteries the baby will undergo a period of hypoxia. This may cause fetal heart changes which may be expressed as any of the following; fetal bradycardia, transient late decelerations, decreased variability or compensatory tachycardia. Once the fit has stopped and maternal hypoxia and acidosis

Table 3.2   Stages of an eclamptic fit

Stage	Length of time in seconds	Possible features
Prodromal or premonitory	10–30	Possible reports of visual disturbances, rapid eye movements, facial twitching and congestion, muscular twitching deepening loss of consciousness
Tonic	10–30	Generalised muscle spasm and rigidity, absent respiration, cyanosis
Tonoclonic	60	Intermittent contraction and relaxation of all body muscles producing convulsive movements The woman is unconscious and may have • stertorous breathing • increased salivation • incontinence of urine and faeces
Final postictal state	A few minutes – several hours	Gradual return to consciousness Spontaneous breathing usually occurs and oxygenation is rarely a problem Respiration may be rapid and deep Possible amnesia of events prior to fit Possible confusion, agitation, lethargy

have been corrected, these changes may resolve. However, other factors such as the stage of gestation and the presence of any intrauterine growth restriction influence the prognosis (Usta and Sibai 1995).

Eclampsia in the postnatal period

After the birth pre-eclampsia will usually resolve as the cause has been removed. However, in the immediate postnatal period pre-eclampsia may initially worsen (Greer in Chamberlain and Steer 2001). Some women may exhibit the signs and symptoms of severe pre-eclampsia for the first time in the postpartum period (Redman 2002). In the study conducted by Douglas and Redman (1994), 44 per cent of fits occurred postnatally. Twelve per cent of cases occurred more than 48 hours after delivery and 2 per cent more than seven days after delivery. Mattar and Sibai (2000) identified 399 women who suffered eclampsia in one medical centre in the USA; 110 (28 per cent) developed postpartum eclampsia. Because pre-eclampsia may initially worsen before resolving, appropriate levels of monitoring should continue for up to 48 hours. Midwives need to be aware of this in order to plan effective postnatal care.

Principles of the immediate management of eclampsia

Once an eclamptic fit has occurred, the attending health professional needs to act promptly and to follow an appropriate action plan. The aim of this book is to focus on management of obstetric emergencies outside the hospital environment. The exact order of actions will depend upon the setting within which the fit takes place. A community midwife may be the first health professional attending a woman at home. It is acknowledged that often they are lone workers who carry a limited amount of equipment. Birth centres or midwifery lead units, although predominantly low-tech environments, may have access to more personnel, resources and equipment. These considerations must be borne in mind when reading the following possible action plan. However, the overriding principles of management remain the same: you must make an assessment of the woman's condition and prioritise actions. At all times the midwife will use personal knowledge and clinical judgement to practise safely within the Midwives Rules and Code of Practice (UKCC 1998). Account will be taken of local trust guidelines.

- Call for medical assistance.
- Follow the principles of resuscitation: Airway, Breathing and Circulation.
- Ensure the safety of the woman.
- Monitor both mother and baby.
- Arrange for immediate transfer to the most appropriate obstetric and medical facility.

Call for medical assistance

A paramedic ambulance needs to be called immediately, giving full details of the situation and address. If you are in the home situation you may consider calling a second midwife or general practitioner to give extra professional assistance. For example, they may assist with setting up equipment, taking observations or supporting relatives.

Follow the principles of resuscitation and ensure safety

Airway

During the eclamptic fit it is very difficult to do anything other than make the environment safe by moving objects such as furniture out of the woman's way and placing towels or anything else appropriate between the woman and hard surfaces. Falls from a bed or couch should be prevented to minimise head injury. As soon as the fit has stopped, it is vitally important to establish an airway and place the woman in the recovery position. Depending upon where the fit takes place, it may be necessary to move the woman in order to give yourself more space to care for her. Because you may be working on your own you need to minimise the risk of damage to yourself and the mother by practising safe handling.

Once the fit has stopped, continue to maintain the woman's safety. As you do this, assess the woman's airway, breathing and colour. It is vitally important to establish an airway; you may need to clear secretions from her mouth as during the fit or in the postfit period she may vomit. Suction can be used if this is available. Place her in the recovery position on her left side to relieve aortocaval compression. It may be necessary to place a wedge such as a towel under her right hip. This position maximises uterine blood flow and venous return to the heart and minimises the risk of aspiration (Jevon and Raby 2001). Assess if the woman has injured herself during the fit; she may have bitten her tongue.

Breathing

According to the ALSO guidelines (1996) in the postfit period spontaneous breathing usually occurs. Ensure that breathing is regular by observing her respiration rate. Respiratory problems may occur if the woman suffers repeated fits. Administer oxygen if available; oxygen at a flow rate of at least ten litres per minute will achieve an inspired oxygen concentration of approximately 90 per cent (Jevon and Raby 2001).

Circulation

Establish that there is a pulse. Observations of maternal blood pressure and of skin colour need to be taken in order continuously to monitor improvement or deterioration in the woman's condition. If equipment is available and personnel have the appropriate training, intravenous cannulation with a large-bore cannula, at least 16-gauge, needs to be undertaken. This will allow administration of intravenous medication. Careful fluid balance is needed to avoid the iatrogenic morbidity associated with fluid overload (Baldwin et al. 2001). The guidelines for the management of severe pre-eclampsia in the CEMD (NICE 2001) recommends fluid intake be restricted to 85ml/h. Advice needs to be sought from the senior obstetrician at the receiving unit for the type of intravenous fluid to be used. Alternatively the cannula can be flushed to maintain patency. If the necessary resources are available, catheterisation can take place and maternal input and output can be documented on a fluid balance chart.

Monitor mother and baby

Level of consciousness

Following the fit the woman's level of consciousness needs to be assessed. This can be carried out using the Glasgow Coma Scale (Harrison and Daly 2001). During the postictal period the woman maybe agitated and confused. Sensory stimulation may provoke or worsen her agitation (Usta and Sibai 1995). She may have no memory about events occurring before the fit. It is very important to continue to talk to the woman and explain all your actions. This will give reassurance and orientate her to what is going on around her.

Abdominal examination

In cases of eclampsia occurring during pregnancy or labour, palpate the tone of the uterus, as one of the complications during an eclamptic fit is the risk of placental abruption and uterine hyperactivity (Barton et al. 1992). As the fetus is at risk of hypoxia as explained earlier, the fetal heart rate should be monitored and documented. Placental abruption may be accompanied by bleeding which may be revealed, concealed or mixed. Eclampsia may be accompanied by disseminated intravascular coagulation. Since this indicates a very serious deterioration in the woman's health, it is essential that signs such as bruising, bleeding from the nose, mouth and cannulation site, the absence of clots in any blood loss, and haematuria are promptly detected and reported.

Arrange for transfer from community into hospital

The local delivery suite needs to be informed of the emergency, and advice needs to be sought from the senior obstetrician, preferably the on-call consultant, as to the most appropriate medication to give and the most appropriate facility for transfer. In many rural areas there may be no choice of facility. However, in urban areas there may be a more appropriate unit to which to transfer an eclamptic woman. Gaining advice from the receiving unit will ensure that the plan of care will be in keeping with the protocols and preferences of the lead obstetrician and anaesthetist. Advice will vary according to the situation: whether the fit continues or is self-limiting, whether the woman is in the antenatal or postnatal period, and the distance needed to travel during transfer.

It is important to establish clearly where the obstetric team will meet you, as this allows staff of the receiving unit to be prepared. Taking an eclamptic woman via accident and emergency is not appropriate and may result in dangerous time-wasting. According to Burnett (1997), eclampsia is rarely seen in emergency departments and staff may not be familiar with eclampsia protocols. Taking the woman directly to the delivery suite will allow for immediate commencement of magnesium sulphate, antihypertensive therapy and monitoring of mother and baby.

If you are the midwife who attends the woman, you do not relinquish care. During the transfer you continue to work with the other health professionals present. Close monitoring of maternal and fetal condition will continue. The transfer of an undelivered woman with eclampsia is hazardous, as the ambulance journey may subject the woman to increased sensory stimulation and precipitate more convulsions (Salha and Walker 1999). Sibai (1990) considers the transport of an eclamptic woman to be particularly dangerous, and therefore further fits must be anticipated and prepared for. Throughout the transfer the regime of airway, breathing and circulation needs to continue.

Medication for eclampsia in the community

Magnesium sulphate has become the drug of choice in the management of eclampsia and has become standard practice in the hospital environment throughout the UK. The CEMD (NICE 2001) recommends giving an intravenous loading dose of 4 g of magnesium sulphate over five to ten minutes followed by a maintenance infusion of 1–2 g/h at the discretion of the consultant in charge. Sources appear to suggest that magnesium sulphate works by reversing the cerebral vasoconstriction (Redman 2002). The assessment of magnesium sulphate is based on the results of a large international multicentre randomised trial that compared magnesium sulphate with diazepam and phenytoin for the management of eclampsia (Eclampsia Trial Collaboration Group 1995). The trial concluded that when compared with diazepam or phenytoin, magnesium sulphate was a more effective hypotensive and anticonvulsant treatment.

However, the evidence base for the treatment of eclampsia in low-tech settings in the UK has not been established. With this consideration in mind, 14 consultant obstetricians throughout the UK were approached for their views regarding the treatment of eclampsia in the community setting. Of the 11 who responded, all reiterated that magnesium sulphate is the optimal management plan for eclampsia. In relation to the emergency management of eclampsia in non-hospital settings, it was recognised that whilst magnesium sulphate may not be currently available, some paramedic teams may carry a diazemules injection (Scott 2004). When respondents were asked about the appropriateness of giving diazemules in an emergency, five consultants felt it reasonable in cases where the fit was witnessed. Two were not convinced that variation from standard practice was indicated and two felt diazemules should not be given. This latter response reflects ALSO guidelines (1996) which caution against attempting to shorten the initial convulsion by using diazemules, on the basis that a 'polypharmacy' approach is not recommended in the treatment of eclampsia as this is likely to confuse the clinical picture. Six consultants considered the intramuscular administration of magnesium sulphate to be an appropriate alternative and easier to administer in the community setting.

In summary, magnesium sulphate is not freely available in a community setting but there may be access to diazemules. However, it is imperative that advice is taken from the senior obstetrician in the receiving unit as to the appropriateness of administering any medications. If medications are used, the midwife needs to be familiar with their administration, dosage and side effects.

Documentation

Documentation will include times of all actions and treatments, and times and names of all other health professionals that attended. It may be difficult to keep a contemporaneous account of the situation. As soon as it is appropriate to do so, documentation needs to be completed. Once the transfer is complete and care has been handed over to the receiving midwife, entries in the records may be made retrospectively. The supervisor of midwives needs to be informed of the situation.

Family support

It cannot be overstated how frightening a fit must be for those who witness it. Anxiety and fear may produce a state of extreme psychological arousal which can interfere with a person's ability to function and to follow directions (Hayes 2000). Family members need a clear explanation of what is happening and the plans for transfer into hospital. Arrangements may need to be made for child care, or for next of kin to be contacted.

Conclusion

This chapter has explored the relationship between the underlying pathophysiology of pre-eclampsia and the signs and symptoms that may occur. The maternal systemic reaction will determine which organ systems are affected, and the pre-eclampsia process will progress at a different rate in different women. The crises that can occur as a result of the pre-eclampsia process have been outlined, and eclampsia has been focused upon. Although the aim of care is to prevent the condition deteriorating into a crisis, cases of eclampsia still occur outside the hospital environment. Community health professionals need, therefore, to keep themselves updated with contemporary knowledge of the condition and have prepared action plans in advance of the emergency arising.

Supervisor of midwives' commentary

Part of the role of a supervisor of midwives is actively to promote a high standard of care and although, as identified in this chapter, eclampsia is relatively uncommon in the UK, midwives need to be vigilant at all ante-natal, intrapartum and postnatal assessments so as to detect early signs and symptoms of pre-eclampsia. The importance of this cannot be over-stated because early intervention with appropriate care can prevent pre-eclampsia progressing to a critical condition.

The majority of community-based midwives and those practising in a low-tech environment are likely to have limited experience of caring for women with severe pre-eclampsia or eclampsia because once the condition has been recognised the mother's care will be transferred to an obstetric unit and the management of care will be dependant upon the severity of her condition. However, any midwife working in the community or birth centre may be faced with the need to deal with fulminating pre-eclampia and eclampsia at any time. It is of extreme importance that (s)he would be able to undertake the management of this emergency as described in the chapter and is required to do so in accordance with Rule 40, Midwives Rules and Code of Practice (UKCC 1998).

Key points

- Call for appropriate help.
- Administer immediate care to ensure the wellbeing of the mother.
- Carry out observations of maternal and fetal wellbeing.
- It is extremely important not to lose sight of the need for informed consent when carrying out any procedure, even during times of crisis.
- Arrange transfer to an obstetric unit for as soon as is appropriate (this will include seeking advice from a senior obstetrician regarding when it is suitable to transfer).
- Travel with the mother in the ambulance.
- If unable to make contemporaneous notes, remember times and the sequence of events then complete record-keeping as soon as possible after the event (Rule 42, Midwives Rules and Code of Practice (UKCC 1998)).
- Inform the on-call supervisor of midwives of the situation and management of the case.

- Keep up to date with both the theoretical and practical management of such cases.

Obstetric commentary

Pre-eclampsia is a multisystem disorder which is unpredictable in its onset, progress and effects on both mother and baby. Sadly, as reported in the confidential enquiries, in some cases there is failure to recognise the condition and/or its seriousness.

The pathogenesis of the disease, described in great length, may appear very detailed, but it would help the reader to understand the basis of the clinical picture of hypertensive disorders with pregnancy.

Women with pre-eclampsia are usually asymptomatic; if symptoms develop they indicate worsening of the condition. Warning symptoms are headaches, flashing lights, nausea and epigastric pains. The latter is the most sinister symptom and should not be ignored. It must be remembered that, even with severe pre-eclampsia, the risk of progressing to eclampsia is only 1 per cent.

The diagnosis of pregnancy-induced hypertension relies on the measurement of blood pressure (BP) and proteinuria, both of which may not be representative. For example, there is still a controversy about how to measure BP. The current view is that the woman should be either sitting or in left lateral position with the sphygmomanometer at the level of the heart. Korotkoff sound V (disappearance of heart sounds) should be used for measurement of diastolic pressure rather than IV (muffling of heart sounds). Automated BP measurement is advocated to ensure consistency. With regard to proteinuria, the diagnosis, if reagents strips are used, may not be accurate as it can be altered with the urine dilution, contamination or infection.

If the condition is complicated by seizures or coma, it would be classified as eclampsia, literally meaning flashing lights. Eclampsia remains a significant cause of maternal mortality. However, the seizures are not often the cause of death but it is the underlying pathology (women with epilepsy seizures have lower mortality rates). Differential diagnosis of other causes of convulsions such as epilepsy, subarachnoid haemorrhage and meningitis should be considered.

Most patients with eclampsia have systolic BPs over 160 mmHg or diastolic BPs over 110 mmHg. However, as described in this chapter, eclampsia can occur with minimally elevated BP. In addition, most patients have signs and symptoms representative of end-organ damage prior to development of seizures; these include headache, visual disturbances, confusion, abdominal pain, proteinuria, oliguria, pulmonary oedema, generalised peripheral oedema, and fetal growth restriction.

Eclampsia is associated with a substantial degree of maternal and neonatal morbidity and mortality because of the associated maternal vascular damage and intrauterine growth restriction, in addition to the risk of iatrogenic preterm delivery.

Eclampsia occurs most commonly during the antepartum period, yet about one third of cases occur during the postpartum period. Although seizures are reported as late as three weeks postpartum, the majority of cases occur in the first postpartum day.

The management of the fit is well described in the chapter and I cannot emphasise too strongly the importance of the resuscitation principles: Airway, Breathing and Circulation. It is essential to monitor the woman's consciousness (Glasgow Conscious Scale) and avoid fluid overloading which can easily happen if careful attention is not paid to accurate fluid balance. Once the seizure has ended and the ABC are secured, you should call for assistance and prepare the patient for transfer to the nearest maternity unit with high-dependency, one-to-one care. Availability of intensive care may also be needed if complicated with pulmonary oedema, adult respiratory distress syndrome, renal failure, coagulopathy or cerebral haemorrhage. If a health professional who is qualified to prescribe and administer intravenous (IV) therapy is available, consider treating repeated successive fits with IV diazemuls and severe hypertension with IV hydralazine.

It must be frightening to find yourself confronted with a fitting woman in an unfamiliar environment. I found the scenario a useful tool for learning how to deal with such a situation in a preplanned way and appreciating the information rather than just memorising it.

Key points

- Hypertensive disease during pregnancy is associated with a substantial degree of maternal and neonatal morbidity and mortality.
- Eclamptic fits may occur without warning symptoms or signs.
- The only cure is the delivery of the fetus.
- In pre-eclampsia, supportive management may be considered in some cases to prolong the pregnancy.
- With eclampsia, it is essential to transfer the woman to a hospital where the appropriate resources and facilities are available. Luckily, most women would have only one convulsion and this should give time for the attendant to organise transfer.
- Inform the obstetric unit. Meanwhile, consider what is available in the setting for dealing with mother and baby awaiting transfer:
  - maintain airway patency (if available, oxygen mask and pulse oximetry);

- automated BP (if available electrocardiogram);
- insert a cannula (take bloods and start IV infusion slowly);
- maintain accurate fluid balance (insert an indwelling urinary catheter);
- assess fetal wellbeing (use Sonicaid).

A problem-based scenario and interactive action planning exercise
Managing fulminating pre-eclampsia in the community

Jane is a 44-year-old who is a gravida 2, para 1. She lives 20 miles away from the nearest hospital. Eight years ago she had an uncomplicated pregnancy and labour. This pregnancy is with a new partner David. On booking at 12 weeks' gestation, Jane's BP was 110/65 and urinalysis showed no abnormalities. During her antenatal visit at 27 weeks' gestation, Jane says that she thinks that she has put on a lot of weight over the past three weeks. She is wearing flip-flops as her ankles and feet are so swollen she cannot get her shoes on. Her BP is 125/80 and urinalysis reveals 1 + protein. Jane is referred to the day assessment unit for investigations and monitoring. Following this her BP recordings become normotensive.

Three days later you are the community midwife on call; Jane is not in your caseload. Jane's partner David phones you. He says that Jane feels nauseous and has a headache.

Write down what action is necessary and why?

Action plan

David's call gives cause for concern as he has mentioned the following signs of pre-eclampsia:

- headache
- nausea.

Jane needs immediate attendance at home. You need to use your own clinical judgement to decide if you call for an ambulance at this time.

On your way to Jane's house mentally rehearse how you will assess Jane's condition.

You arrive at Jane's house. David lets you in saying, 'Jane's not making any sense, she's upstairs in the bathroom being sick and she's got a terrible headache, the worst pain in her life.' As you find Jane, she falls to the floor and both her arms and legs start to jerk violently. She is having a fit.

List the sequence of your immediate actions whilst Jane is fitting and in the time immediately following the fit. Remember you are the health professional who has found Jane, you are on your own and must make decisions.

Possible action plan

- The order of your actions will be different in varying situations. You must make an assessment of the woman's condition and prioritise actions. Remember the principles of Airway, Breathing and Circulation; it is vitally important to establish an airway as soon as you possibly can.
- If not called already, call for a paramedic (ideally trained in obstetrics) ambulance. Can you trust the partner to call whilst you attend Jane? It may be better if you use your mobile phone to dial 999, therefore being assured that accurate information about the situation and the address have been given to ambulance control.
- Consider calling a second midwife or a general practitioner. They may be nearer to Jane's home and may arrive before the paramedics, giving you extra professional support.
- During the fit attend to Jane's safety. You may need to place towels or anything else appropriate between Jane and hard surfaces.
- Once the fit has stopped it may be necessary to move Jane for her own safety.
- Assess the airway. If necessary, establish and maintain the airway. You may have to clear secretions from her mouth.
- Establish if breathing is regular and give oxygen when it is available.
- Place Jane on her side in the recovery position to maintain a patent airway and to prevent aspiration of vomit.
- Maintain continuous observations of skin colour and respiration rate.
- Check circulation and pulse.
- If you have the necessary skills and the equipment is available, insert a large-bore cannula and maintain patency either by flushing the cannula or commencing an intravenous infusion.

→

> →
> - Palpate the tone of the uterus. Is the fundus soft or hard? One of the complications during an eclamptic fit is placental abruption. This may or may not be accompanied by virginal bleeding.
> - Assess fetal heart rate.
> - Check BP when appropriate.
> - Assess Jane' s consciousness level.
> - Establish if Jane has sustained any other injuries.
> - Give David clear information about what is happening.
> - Jane needs to be transferred to hospital immediately. Inform labour ward who can inform the full obstetric emergency team.
> - Discuss the situation with the registrar or consultant on call. Establish the following:
>   - should medications be administered?
>   - necessity for intravenous fluids and type of fluid?
>   - where will the obstetric team meet you?
> - Suggest that David may wish to make arrangements for someone to look after Jane's other child.
> - Maintain a record of events.
> - Whilst waiting for the transfer, decrease sensory stimulation.

Practice review

Take some time out mentally to rehearse what you would do if faced with a woman having an eclamptic fit:

- Who would you call?
- Have you contact numbers readily available?
- In your area what equipment do the obstetric paramedics, midwives and GPs carry?
- Do you know what skills paramedics and GPs have in order to work as an interprofessional team? If not, discuss this with your manager.
- Are you up to date with maternal resuscitation? In the worst-case scenario an eclamptic fit may lead to cardiac arrest which would necessitate the health professional present commencing maternal resuscitation. Jevon and Raby (2001) have written an excellent resource for resuscitation in pregnancy.

References

Action on Pre-eclampsia (2000) *Information Leaflet Pre-eclampsia and Eclampsia: Your Questions Answered.* Action on Pre Eclampsia: Middlesex.

ALSO (Advanced Life Support in Obstetrics) (1996) *Advanced Life Support in Obstetrics Course Syllabus* (3rd edn). American Academy of Family Physicians: Leawood; KS.

Baldwin K, Leighton N A, Kilby M D, Wyldes M, Churchill D and Johanson R B (2001) The West Midlands 'Severe Hypertensive Illness in Pregnancy' (SHIP) Audit, *Hypertension in Pregnancy* **20** (3), 257–68.

Barton J R, Bronstein S K and Sibai B M (1992) Management of the Eclamptic Patient; *The Journal of Maternal–Foetal Medicine* **1**, 313–19.

Brosens I, Robertson, W B and Dixon H G (1967) The Physiological Response of the Vessels of the Placental Bed to Normal Pregnancy, *Journal of Pathology and Bacteriology* **93**, 569–79.

Burnett D (1997) Severe Pre-eclampsia and Eclampsia: A Broad Overview with Discussion of the Nursing Care Required for the Eclamptic Patient; *Accident and Emergency Nursing* **5**, 200–4.

Churchill D and Beevers D G (1999) *Hypertension in Pregnancy*. British Medical Journal Publications: London.

Davey D A and MacGillivray I (1988) The Classification and Definition of the Hypertensive Disorders of Pregnancy, *American Journal of Obstetrics and Gynaecology* **158**, 892–8.

Dekker G and Sibai B (2001) Primary, Secondary, and Tertiary Prevention of Pre-eclampsia, *The Lancet* **357**, 209–14.

Douglas K A and Redman C W (1994) Eclampsia in the United Kingdom, *British Medical Journal* **309**, 1395–9.

Duckett A, Kenny L and Baker P N (2001) Hypertension in Pregnancy, *Current Obstetrics and Gynaecology* **11** (1), 7–14.

Eclampsia Trial Collaboration Group (1995) Which Anticonvulsant for Women with Eclampsia? Evidence from the Collaborative Eclampsia Trial, *The Lancet* **345**, 1455–63.

Greer I (2001) Pregnancy Induced Hypertension. In G Chamberlain and P J Steer (eds), *Turnbull's Obstetrics* (3rd edn). Churchill Livingstone: London.

Hayes N (2000) *Foundations of Psychology* (3rd edn). Thomson Learning: London.

Harrison J and Daly R (2001) *Acute Medical Emergencies A Nursing Guide*. Churchill Livingstone: Edinburgh.

Jevon P and Raby M (2001) *Resuscitation in Pregnancy: A Practical Approach*. Books for Midwives: Oxford.

Katz V L, Farmer R and Kuller J A (2000) Pre-eclampsia into Eclampsia: Toward a New Paradigm, *American Journal of Obstetrics and Gynaecology* **182** (6), 1389–96.

Kean L, Baker P and Edelstone D (2000) *Best Practice in Labour Ward Management*. W B Saunders: Edinburgh.

Khong T Y, De Wolf F, Robertson W B and Brosens I (1986) Inadequate Maternal Vascular Response to Placentation Complicated by Pre-eclampsia and by Small for Gestational Age Infants, *British Journal of Obstetrics and Gynaecology* **93**, 1049–59.

MacDonald S (2002) Pre-eclampsia and Eclampsia. In M Boyle (ed), *Emergencies Around Childbirth: A Handbook for Midwives*. Radcliffe Medical Press: Abingdon.

MacKeigan S (2000) Unveiling Eclampsia, *Canadian Journal of Anesthesiology*, **Summer**, 23–8.

Marsh G N and Renfrew M J (1999) Introduction. In G N Marsh and M J Renfrew (eds), *Community Based Maternity Care*. Oxford University Press: Oxford.

Mattar F and Sibai B (2000) Eclampsia Risk Factors for Maternal Morbidity, *American Journal of Obstetrics and Gynaecology* **19**, 357–60.

McKay K (2000) Biochemical and Blood Tests in Midwifery Practice (1) Pre-eclampsia, *MIDIRS Midwifery Digest* **10** (1), 39–41.

Myers J E and P N Baker (2002) Hypertensive Diseases and Eclampsia, *Current Opinion in Obstetrics and Gynaecology* **14**, 119–25.

NCCWCH (National Collaborating Centre for Women's and Children's Health) (2003) *Antenatal care: Routine Care for the Healthy Pregnant Woman*. Royal College of Obstetricians and Gynaecologists Press: London.

Nelson-Piercy C (2002) *Handbook of Obstetric Medicine* (2nd edn). Martin Dunitz: London.

NICE (National Institute for Clinical Excellence) (2001) *Why Mothers Die 1997–1999; The Confidential Enquiries into Maternal Deaths in the United Kingdom*. Royal College Obstetricians and Gynaecology Press: London.

Redman C (2002) Hypertension. In M de Swiet (ed), *Medical Disorders in Obstetric Practice* (4th edn). Blackwell Science: Oxford.

Redman C W and J M Roberts (1993) Management of Pre-eclampsia, *The Lancet* **341**, 1451–4.

Roberts J M and Cooper D W (2001) Pathogenesis and Genetics of Pre-eclampsia, *The Lancet* **357**, 53–6.

Roberts J M and Lain K Y (2002) Recent Insights into the Pathogenesis of Pre Eclampsia, *Placenta* **23**, 359–72.

Roberts J M and Redman C W (1993) Pre-eclampsia: More than Pregnancy Induced Hypertension, *The Lancet* **341**, 1447–50.

Roberts J M, Taylor R N, Musci T J, Rodgers G M, Hubel C A and McLaughlin M K (1989) Pre-eclampsia: An Endothelial Cell Disorder, *American Journal of Obstetrics and Gynaecology* **161** (3), 1200–4.

Salha O and Walker J (1999) Modern Management of Eclampsia, *Postgraduate Medical Journal* **75**, 78–82.

Scott J (2004) Personal Communication.

Sibai B M (1990) Eclampsia Maternal–Perinatal Outcome in 254 Consecutive Cases; *American Journal of Obstetrics and Gynaecology* **163** (3), 1049–55.

Sidebotham M (2004) NICE Guideline: Antenatal Care under the Microscope, *British Journal of Midwifery* **12** (3), 137–41.

UKCC (United Kingdom Central Council for Nursing, Midwifery and Health Visiting) (1998) *Midwives Rules and Code of Practice*, UKCC: London.

Usta I M and Sibai B M (1995) Emergent Management of Puerperal Eclampsia, *Obstetrics and Gynaecology Clinics of North America* **22** (2), 315–35.

Walker J (1996) Care of the Patient with Severe Pregnancy Induced Hypertension, *European Journal of Obstetrics and Gynaecology and Reproductive Biology* **65**, 127–35.

Walker J (2000) Pre-eclampsia, *The Lancet* **356**, 1260–1.

Walker J (2003) Personal Communication.

Witlin A G (1999) Prevention and Treatment of Eclamptic Convulsions, *Clinical Obstetrics and Gynaecology* **42** (3), 507–18.

4

The Midwife's Management of Shoulder Dystocia

Karen Bates

Introduction

There is no doubt that shoulder dystocia is 'the nightmare scenario'. The realisation that the clock is ticking and, with each passing minute, the fate of this baby lies in your hands is enormous. It is the scenario that has been described as 'wrapping the midwife's heart in terror' (Brauer-Rieke 2000). The impact of the mounting tension building at the point of diagnosing shoulder dystocia is almost impossible to convey through the written word.

Shoulder dystocia is notoriously difficult to prepare for and define with any degree of certainty. It is one thing to be faced with this type of scenario in a consultant unit with assistance more readily available. When it happens in a community setting the midwife may well find herself managing this emergency situation on her own and in the absence of medical help.

For this reason, the midwife at a birth in any setting needs to be ready to manage shoulder dystocia. This presents a paradox since, as midwives, we are desperately trying to maintain the philosophical basis for care as being 'normal'. Approaching every delivery with an attitude of anticipating shoulder dystocia may suggest we relinquish this philosophical basis for care – not at all. The underlying principle for this chapter will be that anticipating shoulder dystocia means that the midwife:

- acknowledges the fact that shoulder dystocia can occur in the absence of risk factors;
- has an understanding of the mechanics of shoulder dystocia;
- is equipped with the knowledge for managing shoulder dystocia;
- establishes where and who the support systems are in the event of shoulder dystocia.

Defining the problem

There is no standard or universally agreed definition for shoulder dystocia. This lack of an accepted definition accounts for a wide variation in reported incidence of between 0.23 and 1.1 per cent of vaginal vertex deliveries (Hope et al. 1998).

There have been several attempts to define the problem (see Table 4.1), but rather than actually 'define' what the midwife is facing as she attempts to deliver the shoulders, 'definitions' are more akin to a 'diagnosis' of the problem.

Many of the definitions involve subjective judgment in relation to just how much difficulty there was in delivering the shoulders. This is problematic since, for example, how much traction is too much traction? Dystocia is a complex clinical scenario and it is vital that the emergency is identified at the earliest opportunity. Once the baby has delivered, further analysis regarding why the shoulders were difficult to deliver can be undertaken. Therefore, although the least recent, Resnik's definition alluding to any difficulty with the delivery of the shoulders is probably the most helpful as it identifies the problem actually faced by the practitioner. The definition may be criticised for being broad, but it enables the midwife promptly to diagnose the problem during the birth and commence management as soon as possible.

The extent of the problem

The incidence of shoulder dystocia is difficult to calculate with any degree of certainty mainly owing to the lack of consensus on the definition, and rates vary between 0.53 per cent of deliveries (Olugbile and Mascarenhas 2000), 0.1 per cent (Christofferson and Rydhstroem 2002) and 1.5 per cent (Ginsberg and Moisidis 2001). Although these rates may not accurately reflect the true picture, they provide an indication.

Table 4.1 Different definitions of shoulder dystocia

Resnik 1980	Manoeuvres other than normal, gentle downward traction are needed to complete the delivery of the anterior shoulder
Smeltzer 1986	Failure of the shoulders spontaneously to traverse the pelvis after the delivery of the head
Kochenour 1991	Failure of the shoulders to cross the pelvic inlet
Lewis and Chamberlain 1990	Shoulder dystocia is when the shoulders remain impacted in the pelvis after delivery of the fetal head. This definition was later refined in the 17th edition of this book (Campbell & Lees 2000): 'Shoulder dystocia means difficult delivery of the shoulders.'
Spong et al. 1995	Prolonged head-to-body delivery time (more than 60 seconds) or the need for ancillary obstetric manoeuvres
Gibb 1995	Gibb defined three degrees of shoulder dystocia: • A tight squeeze of a big baby with the normal mechanism of rotation present • Unilateral dystocia where the posterior shoulder has entered the pelvis but the anterior is stuck above the symphysis pubis • Bilateral dystocia where both shoulders are arrested above the pelvic brim
ALSO 2000	Shoulder dystocia is the impaction of the anterior shoulder against the symphysis pubis after the fetal head has been delivered, and occurs when the breadth of the shoulders is greater than the biparietal diameter of the head

Because of the associated morbidity and mortality to be outlined shortly, even the lowest estimate is significant.

Shoulder dystocia is one of those complications of childbearing which often makes sense 'after the event'. The predisposing factors take on a different meaning when shoulder dystocia is confirmed. For example a 'long' first stage can occur in any delivery; it takes on a different significance in a case of shoulder dystocia. This is where the supervisor of midwives plays a pivotal role in supporting clinical decisions made by the midwife who, at the point of delivery, will not have the benefit of hindsight to know an eventual outcome.

Risk factors

The single most significant risk factor which persists throughout the literature related to shoulder dystocia would appear to be birth-weight (Christofferson and Rydhstroem 2002, Nocon 2000, Bofill et al. 1997).

The incidence of shoulder dystocia in relation to birth-weight increases dramatically as follows:

- 2.5–4 kg incidence of shoulder dystocia is between 0.3 and 1 per cent of deliveries,
- 4–4.5 kg incidence is between 5 and 7 per cent,
- More than 4.5 kg incidence is between 8 and 10 per cent (ALSO 2000).

Birth-weight, by its very definition can only be confirmed at the time of birth. Estimating fetal weight during pregnancy is an inexact science, subject to observer subjectivity. Ultrasound estimation of fetal weight can often be inaccurate, and can therefore be unhelpful (Olugbile and Mascarenhas 2000). In addition to this, the larger the fetus, the more inaccurate ultrasound proves to be (Hope et al. 1998). A study by Benson et al. (1987) found that prediction of macrosomia by ultrasound scan was correct in only 47 per cent of cases. Clements (2002) documents a 15 per cent error estimating fetal weights in the larger babies.

Of course, the midwife will be using other signs and features in order to make clinical judgments, namely abdominal examination and palpation, and the studies cited above would suggest that practitioners should not rely solely on technology to validate clinical findings.

Other risk factors include diabetes because of the risk of fetal macrosomia. However, a risk factor of diabetes will only predict 55 per cent of cases of shoulder dystocia (Acker et al. 1985). Approximately 47 per cent of all shoulder dystocia will occur in infants weighing less than 4 kg. ALSO (2000) puts the figure at over 50 per cent.

Maternal obesity has been identified as a risk factor for shoulder dystocia (Olugbile and Mascarenhas 2000, Sama and Iffy 1998). This factor presents the midwife with additional problems. Assessment of fetal size is very difficult where a woman is obese. The midwife may then request an ultrasound scan to estimate fetal size, only to find comment about the difficulty in obtaining an accurate estimate because of inter-vening maternal adipose tissue. At the point of delivery when the woman is required to adopt different positions to expedite the delivery, an obese woman can find it very difficult to manoeuvre herself into these posi-tions, thus delaying the whole process.

Excessive weight gain during pregnancy has been suggested as a risk factor in anticipating shoulder dystocia (Bennett 1999, Olugbile and Mascarenhas 2000). However, weighing women during the antenatal period has been discontinued as a routine procedure. In these instances it is vital for the midwife to 'listen' to what the woman is saying about her weight gain, and alarm bells should be sounding if the woman is describing weight gain in excess of 13.5 kg during pregnancy (Sama and Iffy 1998). Maternal birth-weight (Klebanhoff et al. 1985) has been iden-tified as being significant enough for midwives to be asking a woman at the booking interview.

Multiparity, as a risk factor, will undoubtedly provide some 'clues' as to how this labour may progress, because a practitioner should be able to access a previous record. However, a previous history can only be helpful if there is an accurate picture of the previous labour; because of the lack of consensus related to 'defining' shoulder dystocia, it may not have been identified in previous labours. Inasmuch as multiparity itself is a risk factor in shoulder dystocia, once again the evidence is not clear and there appears to be a difference of opinion (Toohey et al. 1995, Glynn and Olah 1994, Lewis et al. 1998).

Recognition of the problem

During the first stage of labour, progress may be slow. However, slow progress in first stage of labour is not always helpful as a predictor (Olugbile & Mascarenhas 2000). Indeed, how do we define 'slow' progress? This varies from midwife to obstetrician, from one maternity unit in the country to another. Once again it is part of the jigsaw that may well fit with the confirmation of shoulder dystocia 'after' the event and with the benefit of hindsight.

A prolonged second stage (Bahar 1996, Glynn and Olah 1994) may indicate shoulder dystocia, although once again some studies suggest that this is not always a helpful predictor (Olugbile and Mascarenhas

2000, McFarland at al 1996, Kees et al. 2001). From my personal experience, I have found that where there has been a delay in descent of the fetal head, in the presence of adequate uterine activity during a multiparous labour, it has been due to either an occipito posterior labour or shoulder dystocia. Conversely, I have also experienced shoulder dystocia where there has been a particularly rapid delivery of the baby.

At the point of delivery, shoulder dystocia is usually characterised by a tortuously slow delivery of fetal head, face and chin. Often the face delivers up to the bridge of the fetal nose and the midwife finds herself having to 'peel' the perineum over the rest of the face until the chin finally escapes. Once this point is reached, the fetal head retracts and recoils against the maternal perineum and burrows right back into the maternal tissue. Often there is no restitution because the shoulders have not been able to complete the descent through the pelvis and therefore the normal mechanism of labour is halted.

Under normal circumstances, the anterior shoulder will escape under the pubic arch. This will occur either spontaneously or with the midwife facilitating delivery with downward traction. It is at this point that the midwife recognises that she is unable to complete this manoeuvre and must institute some other manoeuvre to facilitate delivery of the shoulders.

The midwife must resist the urge to maintain traction on the fetal head and encourage the woman to stop 'actively' bearing down with the contractions. This is best done by encouraging the woman to 'Puff, puff, blow! Puff, puff, blow!'

Potential sequelae

The Confidential Enquiry into Stillbirths and Deaths in Infancy 5th Annual Report (CESDI 1998) suggests that one would expect a previously healthy fetus to survive a period of cerebral hypoxia of five minutes or less. Therefore, time is of the essence if neurological complications are to be avoided or minimised.

Erb's palsy or obstetric brachial plexus palsy (OBPP) has increasingly become the subject of litigation (Clements 2002). OBPP is believed to be linked with excessive traction applied to the fetal head. Stirrat and Taylor (2002) provide an excellent critique of the literature in relation to this link. Having examined arguments and counter-arguments, they conclude that 'downward and lateral traction in an attempt to free the anterior shoulder in the presence of shoulder dystocia is the *most*

likely cause of damage to the anterior brachial plexus during birth'. They acknowledge that there are unanswered questions about shoulder dystocia and OBPP in relation to defining shoulder dystocia and the subsequent reporting of OBPP. In particular, the conflict suggested by Limb (2002) between what is **recorded** in relation to the delivery of the shoulders and the *fact* of difficulty in delivering the shoulders.

Other fetal/neonatal outcomes include musculoskeletal injuries, namely fractured humerus or clavicle, although these types of fractures have been noted in spontaneous deliveries in the absence of shoulder dystocia (Nocon 2000).

The psychological trauma of an emergency such as shoulder dystocia on the parents can not be underestimated. Maternal complications include postpartum haemorrhage and genital tract trauma (including anal sphincter and mucosal injury). Uterine rupture is a potential complication, particularly if fundal pressure is used (Harris 1984). Fundal pressure will also exacerbate neurological and musculoskeletal damage in the fetus (Gross, Sokol et al. 1987).

Managing shoulder dystocia

The mnemonic of HELPERRS given below provides one example of a guide for practice. It must be acknowledged that not all practitioners will find mnemonics helpful and will spend time trying to remember what each letter stands for! I have observed this on a number of occasions during emergency scenario workshops attended by post-registration midwives. However, the value is that it does provide structure for dealing with a scenario which, by the very nature of its urgency, can create disordered thought. The more a midwife is given the opportunity to rehearse the structure for dealing with shoulder dystocia, the more she is likely to recall the steps to follow more readily:

Help
Evaluate need for episiotomy
Legs into McRoberts
Pressure (suprapubic)
Enter (hand enters vagina and internal rotational manoeuves are attempted)
Remove (the baby's posterior arm)
Roll (the woman on to 'all fours' (ALSO 2000))
Start all over again.

Figure 4.1 represents the steps required for managing shoulder dystocia at the point of diagnosing it. These are then discussed in greater detail.

Help

The help for which the midwife is calling must obviously be appropriate to the situation. In a home setting or stand-alone birth centre, it is perfectly reasonable to assume that the help being requested is a second midwife or a general practitioner. Within a home setting, the midwife can not be expected to call obstetric help for attendance. However, she must be in a position to request urgent paramedic assistance so that the woman may be transferred into an environment where obstetric help is available. This will form part of the midwife's anticipatory action. If she assumes that shoulder dystocia can occur in *any* delivery regardless of risk factors, she will ensure that she has some method of calling for paramedic assistance and that the method she is using, for example mobile phone, is serviceable. Midwives are often covering community areas with which they are unfamiliar, so need to have prepared themselves for giving ambulance control some idea of their location.

The issue of episiotomy

The issue of when the midwife should perform an episiotomy tends to create debate amongst midwives themselves, as well as between midwives and obstetricians. There is a school of thought which suggests that it should be carried out at this point rather than later, but, on the other hand, if the McRoberts manœuvre is successful there may not be a requirement for an episiotomy. It must be made clear that the reason a midwife will be carrying out this procedure will be to give her room to carry out more invasive manoeuvres later. It will not *resolve* the shoulder dystocia.

Whenever episiotomy is carried out, there is no doubt that this procedure will be difficult. The head is burrowing back into the perineum and it is almost impossible to insert fingers into the vagina, let alone the blade of a pair of scissors. The perineum will be thick, and there is no possibility of infiltration with a local anaesthetic. In some respects it may be more prudent to attempt the less invasive manoeuvres prior to performing an episiotomy, rather than risk possible injury to the practitioner or fetus in carrying out an episiotomy at this time.

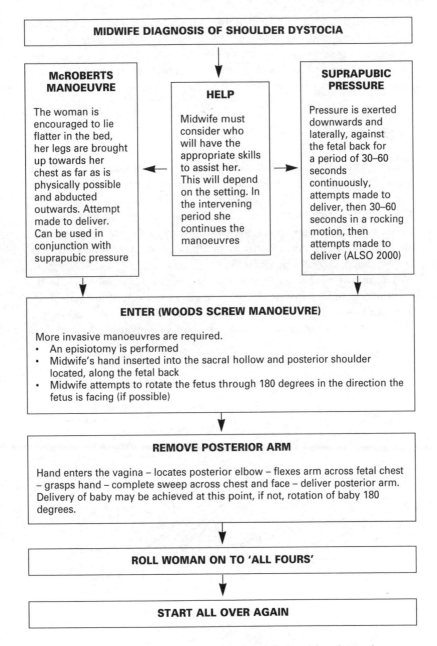

Figure 4.1 Flow chart: managing of shoulder dystocia

The decision to undertake an episiotomy must continue to rest with the midwife at the point of delivery. Whatever the midwife's decision, the contemporaneous records need to reflect his/her evaluation for the need to undertake an episiotomy. If one is not carried out, the records should provide a clear rationale as to why this clinical decision was made.

Legs

Named after William McRoberts, whose name was given to this manoeuvre in the 1950s, the McRoberts manoeuvre is simple, non-invasive and effective as a first response to shoulder dystocia (Figure 4.2). This alters the functional relationships between the pelvic diameters and the diameters of fetal structures. It also reverses almost all of the factors tending to cause shoulder dystocia created by the dorsal lithotomy position (Clements 2002, Coates 1995).

The midwife is going to require assistance for this manoeuvre. In the home environment this could be provided by the birthing partner, a second midwife or the paramedic. The woman herself can adopt this position. If the woman is standing, she can be encouraged to adopt a

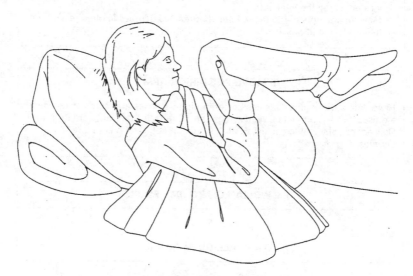

Figure 4.2   McRoberts manoeuvre

squatting position. If she is on the bed, she should be encouraged to bring her buttocks to the edge of the bed, lie flat with her knees brought right up to her chest and opened out as far as she can physically manage. This position is similar to a lithotomy position, but much more exaggerated. The lithotomy position may not provide the degree of abduction and adduction that McRoberts will provide. Gonik et al. (1989) compared the lithotomy position with McRoberts under laboratory conditions and consistently found that there was less force needed to deliver the fetal shoulders when McRoberts was used.

As the woman is encouraged into the McRoberts position, the sacral promontory flattens and the maternal lumbar spine is straightened. This causes the anterior shoulder of the fetus to be elevated and the fetal spine to be flexed (Smeltzer 1986). The posterior shoulder pushes over the sacrum and into the pelvis. The symphysis pubis is rotated superiorly by approximately eight centimetres, which brings the plane of the inlet perpendicular to the maximum maternal expulsive forces (Coates 1997). The midwife should attempt delivery. If there is no advance of the fetal shoulders, the midwife should consider whether the woman could lay any flatter and draw her legs any further upwards and outwards. Delivery should be attempted a second time. If unsuccessful, she should consider the next steps.

The condition symphysis pubis dysfunction may present the midwife with a dilemma, as under normal circumstances the McRoberts position would be contraindicated. It must still be used if possible, but the follow-up of the woman in the postnatal period to assess any exacerbation of the condition is necessary and care should be planned accordingly.

Suprapubic pressure

Suprapubic pressure is an external manoeuvre used to dislodge the anterior shoulder from above the symphysis pubis and reduce the bisacromial diameter (Figure 4.3). Once again, the midwife is going to require assistance from a second midwife. If a paramedic is present, or if there is a birthing partner, the midwife can explain what assistance is required.

Undertaking suprapubic pressure

1   The heel of the hand is placed just above the symphysis pubis and ideally alongside the fetal back. The rationale for this is that if pressure

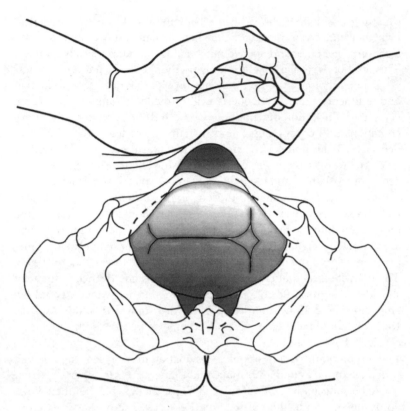

Figure 4.3   Suprapubic pressure

is exerted in the direction the fetus is facing, there is more likelihood of adducting the fetal shoulders and reducing the bisacromial diameter.

2   A second midwife or the paramedic 'under direction' applies pressure against the fetal back, downwards and laterally. The rationale for this is that the anterior shoulder can be dislodged into the transverse diameter, so that it may enter the brim and descend into the pelvis.

3   Initially pressure should be applied continuously for 30–60 seconds and then delivery attempted. If this is not successful then pressure should be applied in a rocking motion for 30–60 seconds (also known as Rubin I manoeuvre) followed again by an attempt at delivery (ALSO 2000, Hinshaw 2003).

Suprapubic pressure can and should be used in conjunction with the McRoberts manoeuvre. The person undertaking this manoeuvre may need to negotiate the woman's legs, but it can be used quite successfully with McRoberts. It can also be used with the more invasive manoeuvres described below.

Fundal pressure should be avoided. It will only serve to impact the shoulder more firmly above the symphysis pubis, and there is a risk of increased damage to the brachial plexus nerves and a risk to the mother of uterine rupture (Gross, Shime et al. 1987).

Enter vagina

If the above manoeuvres are unsuccessful, more invasive manoeuvres will be necessary. It is reasonable to suggest that it is at this point that an episiotomy should be attempted. An episiotomy is not going to release the shoulders but it will provide the midwife with room to insert her hand inside the vagina. It has become very evident to me, as I talk with qualified midwives on this subject, that there is a high level of anxiety related to performing an episiotomy during shoulder dystocia deliveries. It has to be acknowledged that this is a very difficult procedure. In the first instance, the midwife has a limited view of the area where she is to perform the episiotomy because of the head being in the way and the vagina seemingly 'full' of fetal neck. The perineum is thick as it is not being stretched and thinned as usual by the presenting part. These difficulties cannot and should not be underestimated as the midwife is making her decision to perform an episiotomy. Once the episiotomy is undertaken, the midwife's hand is inserted into the vagina to carry out internal manoeuvres.

Internal manoeuvres can create confusion, resulting in high anxiety levels for the midwife as s(he) struggles to remember which aspect of which shoulder needs to be accessed. It does not help when there is a variation in the literature in how these internal manoeuvres are presented.

Woods applied principles of physics to the management of shoulder dystocia (1943) and it is those principles which, once recognised and understood, enable any midwife to adapt the process of manually manoeuvring the fetal shoulders out of the obstruction, through the body of the pelvis and towards the outlet.

After delivery of the head, Woods (1943) likened the shoulders of the

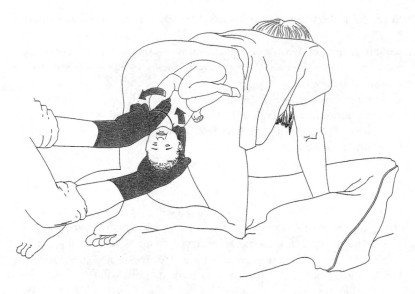

Figure 4.4   Woods manoeuvre

fetus to the 'longitudinal section of a screw engaged in three threads, the pubic thread, the promontory thread and the coccyx thread'. Pulling on the fetal head would be antagonistic to the principle of how a screw works. Applying continued traction on the fetus would be pulling against the threads, rather than enabling the shoulders to negotiate them. Woods describes applying simultaneous pressure to the fetal buttocks with the external hand – not to be confused with fundal pressure – and two fingers internally on the anterior aspect of the posterior shoulder and rotating gently in the direction of the fetal back (Figure 4.4). The shoulders are rotated through 180 degrees until the impacted anterior shoulder is released to become the posterior shoulder. There is a theoretical possibility that applying pressure in this direction could increase the bisacromial diameter by abducting the shoulders (Coates 1997). ALSO (2000) describes the application of pressure against the posterior aspect of the posterior shoulder, which has the effect of adducting the shoulders and reducing the bisacromial diameter.

In the Rubin manoeuvre (1964) the midwife is attempting to access the anterior shoulder. Pressure is applied to the posterior aspect of the anterior shoulder. The rationale in this instance is to reduce the bisacromial diameter of the shoulders and push them into the oblique diameter, out of the anteroposterior diameter in which they are stuck.

Both of these manoeuvres can be used very effectively with suprapubic pressure. Indeed the reality of managing the situation is that any combination involving the Woods or Rubin screw technique may be applied in order to obtain the principle objectives of reducing the bisacromial diameters and enabling the shoulders to negotiate key landmarks and threads of the pelvis.

Remove the posterior arm

In some instances, these rotational manoeuvres may be unsuccessful, and Swartz and Dixon (1958) concluded that removal of the posterior arm was a safe procedure. The midwife's hand is inserted into the vagina, in front of the fetus (Figure 4.5). Pressure is applied to the antecubital fossa, which helps flexion of the arm across the fetal chest. As it flexes, the midwife is able to grasp the hand and bring it out over the face. Once the posterior arm is delivered, the anterior shoulder should disempact and delivery can continue. If this does not happen, rotating the fetus through 180 degrees will unlock the obstruction and complete the delivery.

Roll onto 'all fours'

It may not be the 'all fours' position per se that will facilitate delivery, but rather the movement into the 'all fours' position. Some studies suggest that this position actually maximises pelvic diameters and provides more room along the sacral curve for insertion of the hand (Gaskin 1988, McLean 1989). However, changing into the 'all fours' position may not be easy. The woman will have a fetal head stuck between her legs, she may be a very large lady, tired from her labour and just refuse to move! Once the woman is on 'all fours', it is virtually impossible to undertake effective suprapubic pressure. All these factors need to be taken into account when discussing the feasibility of such actions.

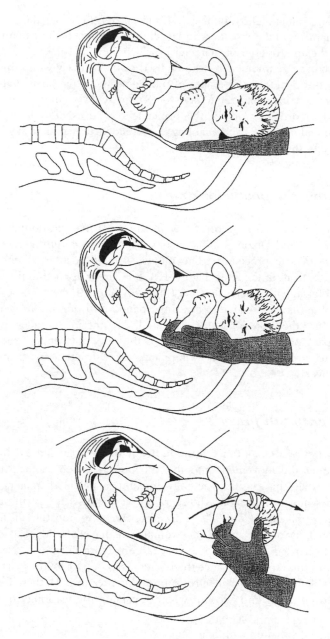

Figure 4.5   Removal of posterior arm

Start all over again

During the journey to hospital and in the absence of obstetric aid, the midwife should continue with the above manoeuvres with the assistance of the paramedic. There is every reason to suspect that the neonate will need some degree of resuscitation. Chapter 7 provides guidance on neonatal resuscitation in the community and during transfer, and on managing the difficult situation when the neonatal outcome is poor. The paediatric team as well as the obstetric team should be alerted to the imminent arrival at hospital via ambulance control and should be standing by to provide the necessary support as appropriate. The midwife may also need to anticipate postpartum haemorrhage, which can be a complication of this emergency situation.

Conclusion

There is no doubt that shoulder dystocia brings with it many ifs and buts, many maybes and howevers. One only needs to read the early part of this chapter to recognise the inherent difficulties in anticipating and defining shoulder dystocia. There seem to be more uncertainties than certainties.

I have often felt that shoulder dystocia is one thing in childbirth that appears so very clear 'after' the event. So many of the pieces of the jigsaw can fit when we know there was an outcome of shoulder dystocia, and yet they could just as easily apply to uncomplicated childbirth scenarios.

This chapter has attempted to demonstrate that as long as the midwife has an understanding of the mechanics of shoulder dystocia and is clear about the principles of dealing with it, it is possible to adapt a variation of recognised manoeuvres until such time as the baby is delivered or she is able to access senior obstetric help.

Supervisor of midwives' commentary

Shoulder dystocia can happen with any delivery and in the absence of predisposing factors. With this in mind, midwives should be prepared to face such a situation with any delivery they attend. Because the life of the fetus depends upon timely and effective management, diagnosis needs be made promptly. As this chapter identifies, shoulder dystocia simply means difficulty in delivering the shoulders, and when a midwife makes this clinical diagnosis, (s)he should not be criticised for 'overreaction'. Midwives need to be supported in their decision at the point of initiating manoeuvres to deliver the shoulders. It is not for another person, even if in the room, to suggest that it could not possibly have been shoulder dystocia. Supervisory support is essential in creating an environment in which midwives feel their clinical decision was appropriate and correct under the circumstances that faced them at the time.

Recently, midwives and obstetricians have been criticised for failing to carry out the standard manoeuvres required when shoulder dystocia has been diagnosed (NHS Litigation Authority 2003). It is essential that midwives keep themselves up to date with their local policies and procedures, and attend workshops and seminars in order to practise the skills needed to manage shoulder dystocia in the relative safety of the classroom.

Key points in managing shoulder dystocia

- Call for appropriate help as soon as shoulder dystocia is suspected.
- Resist the urge to apply traction, and stop the woman from pushing. Fundal pressure is not recommended.
- Implement manoeuvres.
- Record accurately the sequence of events – this should include all manoeuvres carried out and by whom, and also which shoulder is anterior initially.
- Attend updates and training.

Obstetric commentary

Shoulder dystocia is a well-known obstetric emergency and, as explained in this chapter, the incidence depends on the definition used. A realistic and practical definition would include any difficulty in extracting the shoulders after delivering the head. The chapter has addressed the lack of clear definitions, highlighting the contradictions as well as the controversy in the literature.

There is a definite link between the incidence of shoulder dystocia and the size of the baby. Ultrasound-estimated fetal weight certainly has its limitations, but I still believe that it is more accurate than clinical examination (especially in the obese woman). More than one reading can be helpful and the 90th centile, rather than the actual weight, can be taken as the reference for a macrosomic baby at any stage of the pregnancy. A triad of obesity, diabetes and post-dates was noted to have a higher incidence of macrosomic babies and shoulder dystocia (Spellacy et al. 1985).

Some medico-legal experts may consider the presence of multiple risk factors of having a macrosomic baby as a reliable predictor of shoulder dystocia. This is not absolutely true as brachial plexus injury in these cases, if the delivery is managed properly, can not be considered as negligent practice. No study has yet found a single factor or a combination of factors that can be considered as a reliable predictor and, as the chapter has indicated, half the cases occur in babies weighing less than 4000 g. Inappropriate management, excessive traction or fundal pressure, however, would not be defendable.

Traumas to the baby that occur with shoulder dystocia are mainly due to nerve fibres/plexus stretch or damage and are usually transitional and leave no permanent effect. An interesting study of the cost-effectiveness of elective Caesarean section, where the estimated fetal weight was over 4500 g, showed that to prevent one permanent brachial plexus injury, more than 3500 Caesarean sections would have to be performed (Rouse et al. 1996).

The description of the delivery and the different manoeuvres needed to achieve it is quite clear and comprehensive. The chapter is bursting with useful information, practical tips and up-to-date references, and is an excellent overview of such an uncommon but serious scenario which may face any health professional attending birth.

The issue of episiotomy is undoubtedly a controversial and thought-provoking step in the management, and it was a challenging one for me. I was led to believe that an early episiotomy is of great value and delaying it is considered inappropriate, so I had to look into the literature to support my beliefs with the evidence. To my surprise, it seems that most, but not all, authors would recommend an early episiotomy (with the McRoberts manoeuvre and the suprapubic pressure), but none of them provide convincing evidence for its benefit at this stage.

Trauma to the mother is also increased with shoulder dystocia: postpartum haemorrhage is reported in two out of three cases and there is an increase in the incidence of extended vaginal tears and fourth degree perineal tears (Benedetti & Gabbe 1978)

Key points

- Shoulder dystocia is one of the obstetric emergencies.
- Simulated training workshops are useful, but drill is not a substitute for clinical experience or judgement.

- It can not be predicted with any degree of reliability but may be suspected in the following cases:
  - history of diabetes, previous large baby
  - clinically large for dates or estimated weight above 90th centile
  - obesity, post-dates
  - prolonged second stage.
- Disimpacting the anterior shoulder is the mainstay of the management which can be achieved by the following:
  - McRoberts manoeuvre
  - suprapubic pressure
  - large episiotomy (may not be necessary at this stage!).
- Other manoeuvres would entail inserting a hand into the vagina to deliver the posterior shoulder and would require an episiotomy.
- Avoid excessive traction on the neck and do not apply fundal pressure.
- After appropriate resuscitation, examine the baby for evidence of trauma.
- Remember to write contemporaneous delivery notes that should not be just blatantly self-serving.
- Caesarean section or early induction of labour are not justifiable in suspected large for dates.

A problem-based scenario and interactive action planning exercise
A case of shoulder dystocia whilst on call

You are a community midwife. You are covering a colleague's community area whilst she attends a home delivery as a second midwife on call. You receive a call to attend Sally, a 23-year-old, at term with her second baby. The message you receive is that she thinks she is probably in labour.

When you arrive at the home, it is clear that she is in advanced labour, there are clear external signs of full dilation with a visible vertex and you recognise the need to plan for a delivery at home. Her husband Allen is with her and their two-year-old daughter is staying away from home with her grandparents.

Sally adopts a hands and knees position as the head emerges extremely slowly. The contraction stops at the point of delivery up to the bridge of the fetal nose. You find yourself having to push the perineum over the face and chin, and the head burrows back into the maternal tissue.

The next contraction builds up, there is no restitution and no advancement of the shoulders. Lateral flexion by you confirms no advancement of the shoulders.

Write down what immediate action is necessary and why.

Your plan of care should include the following:

- You diagnose shoulder dystocia because you recognise the need to apply other manoeuvres to complete delivery of the shoulders.
- Someone needs to contact a paramedic ambulance – you are aware that the midwife who should be with you is already in attendance at another birth. Consider calling a general practitioner. Can you trust the partner to call whilst you attend Sally? It may be better if you make the call as you are then assured that accurate information about the situation has been transmitted.
- This is not the area you normally cover – do you know where you are? Is your mobile phone battery fully charged with enough talk time or is there a telephone in the house?

You have called for help – the GP and paramedic ambulance are on their way. What is your next course of action?

- Sally is already in a hands and knees position – consider encouraging her to adopt a squatting position which is effectively a McRoberts manoeuvre. Can you complete delivery of the baby?
- You need to be able to undertake suprapubic pressure so you need to assist Sally to adopt a position where this is possible, in other words, on her back in the McRoberts position. Sally and Allen can help you with her legs. Undertake suprapubic pressure. Can you complete delivery of the baby?

Sally has tried squatting and you have tried to deliver the baby. There is no advance of the shoulders. She is now on her back in a McRoberts position. Allen is helping her to hold her legs up.

You have tried suprapubic pressure. What is your next course of action?

- You need to move to more invasive manoeuvres to facilitate this delivery, which means inserting your hand into the vagina. Have you been able to perform an episiotomy?
- Insert your hand into the vagina and locate the posterior shoulder. Which way do you need to rotate this fetus? What are the principles of care? You know that the shoulders need to negotiate the three threads of the 'screw' – the symphysis pubis, the sacral promontory and the coccyx. If you apply pressure to the posterior aspect of the posterior shoulder, you increase the adduction and therefore narrow the bisacromial diameters.

You have managed to perform an episiotomy and have attempted the screw manoeuvres, but this manoeuvre was unsuccessful. What is your next course of action?

- You need to attempt to remove and deliver the posterior arm. Sally had adopted the 'all fours' position during this labour. The 'all fours' position can facilitate this manoeuvre – consider the use of this position.
- Insert your hand into the vagina posteriorally – locate the posterior arm and elbow – flex the arm across the front of the fetal chest – grasp the forearm and bring the arm across the chest and face.
- Try to deliver. You may need to undertake a rotational manoeuvre of 180 degrees to complete the delivery.
- Try all fours. If she is already in this position, move her around onto her back – movement may dislodge the anterior shoulder.

References

Acker D B, Sachs B P and Friedman E A (1985) Risk Factors for Shoulder Dystocia, *Obstetrics Gynaecology* **66**, 762–8.

ALSO (Advanced Life Support in Obstetrics) UK (2000) *Course Syllabus UK.* ALSO: Newcastle upon Tyne.

Bahar A M (1996) Risk Factors and Fetal Outcomes in Cases of Shoulder Dystocia Compared With Normal Deliveries of a Similar Birth Weight, *British Journal of Obstetrics and Gynaecology* **103**, 868–72.

Benedetti T J and Gabbe S G (1978) Shoulder Dystocia. A complication of Fetal Macrosomia and Prolonged Second Stage of Labor with Midpelvic Delivery, *Obstetrics Gynaecology* (Nov) **52** (5), 526–9.

Bennett B B (1999) Shoulder Dystocia: An Obstetric Emergency, *Obstetrics and Gynaecology Clinics of North America* **26** (3), 445–58.

Benson C B, Doubilet P M and Saltzman D H (1987) Sonographic Determination of Fetal Weights in Diabetic Pregnancies, *American Journal of Obstetrics and Gynaecology* **156**, 441–4.

Bofill J A, Rust O A, Devidas M, Roberts W E, Morrison J C and Martin J N (1997) Shoulder Dystocia and Operative Vaginal Delivery, *Journal of Maternal–Fetal Medicine* **6** (4), 220–4.

Brauer-Rieke G (2000) Shoulder Dystocia: The Event That Wraps a Midwife's Heart in Cold Terror, *Midwifery Today with International Midwife* **Issue 55**, 28–9.

Campbell S and Lees C (2000) *Obstetrics by Ten Teachers 17th Edition*. Edward Arnold: London.

CESDI (Confidential Enquiry into Stillbirths and Deaths in Infancy) *5th Annual Report* (1998) Maternal and Child Health Research Consortium.

Christofferson M and Rydhstroem H (2002) Shoulder Dystocia and Brachial Plexus Injury: A Population-Based Study, *Gynaecological and Obstetric Investigation* **53** (1), 42–7.

Clements R V (2002) Editorial: Shoulder Dystocia, *Clinical Risk* **8**, 215–7.

Coates T (1995) Shoulder Dystocia. Ch. 4 in J Alexander, V Levy and S Roch (eds), *Aspects of Midwifery Practice*. Macmillan: Basingstoke.

Coates T (1997) Manoeuvres for the Relief of Shoulder Dystocia, *Modern Midwife* (Sept) **7** (9) 15–9.

Gaskin I M (1988) Shoulder Dystocia: Controversies in Management, *Birth Gazette* **5**, 14.

Gibb D (1995) Clinical Focus: Shoulder Dystocia: The Obstetrics, *Clinical Focus* **1**, 49–54.

Ginsberg N A and Moisidis C (2001) How to Predict Recurrent Shoulder Dystocia, *American Journal of Obstetrics and Gynaecology* **184** (7), 1427–30.

Glynn M and Olah K S (1994) The Management of Shoulder Dystocia, *British Journal of Midwifery* **2** (3) 108–12.

Gonik B, Allen R and Sorab J (1989) Objective Evaluation of the Shoulder Dystocia Phenomenon: Effect of Maternal Pelvic Orientation on Force Reduction, *Obstetrics and Gynaecology* **74** (1), 44–8.

Gross S J, Shime J and Forrine D (1987) Shoulder Dystocia: Predictors and Outcome: A Five Year Review, *American Journal of Obstetrics and Gynaecology* **26** (2) 334–6.

Gross T, Sokol R, Williams T and Thompson K (1987) Shoulder Dystocia, A Fetal-Physician Risk, *American Journal of Obstetrics and Gynaecology* **156**, 882–4.

Harris B A (1984) Shoulder Dystocia, *Clinical Obstetrics and Gynaecology* **27** (1) 106–11.

Hinshaw K (2003) Shoulder Dystocia. In R Johanson, C Cox, K Grady and C Howell, *Managing Obstetric Emergencies and Trauma: The MOET Course Manual.* RCOG Press: London.

Hope P, Breslin S and Lamont L (1998) Fatal Shoulder Dystocia: A Review of 56 Cases Reported to the Confidential Enquiry into Stillbirths and Deaths in Infancy, *British Journal of Obstetrics and Gynaecology* **105**, 1256–61.

Kees S, Margalit V and Schiff E (2001) Features of Shoulder Dystocia in a Busy Obstetric Unit, *Journal of Reproductive Medicine* **46** (6), 583–8.

Klebanhoff M A, Mills J L and Berendes H W (1985) Mother's Birthweight as a Predictor of Macrosomia, *American Journal of Obstetrics and Gynaecology* **153**, 253–7.

Kochenour N K (1991) Intrapartum Obstetric Emergencies, *Critical Care Clinics* **7** (4), 851–8.

Lewis D F, Edwards M S, Asrat T et al. (1998) Can Shoulder Dystocia be Predicted?, *Journal of Reproductive Medicine* **43** (8), 654–8.

Lewis T L T and Chamberlain G V P (1990) *Obstetrics by Ten Teacher 15th Edition.* Edward Arnold: London.

Limb C (2002) [A Child] v The Countess of Chester Hospitals NHS Trust, *Clinical Risk* **8**, 2225–6.

McFarland M B, Langer O, Piper J M and Berkus M D (1996) Perinatal Outcome and the Type and Number of Manoeuvres in Shoulder Dystocia, *International Journal of Obstetrics and Gynaecology* **55**, 219–24.

McLean M T (1989) Managing Shoulder Dystocia, *Midwifery Today* **12**, 24–5.

NHS Litigation Authority (2003) Summary of Substandard care in cases of obstetric brochial plexus injury, *A Journal for Practising Clinicians* **2**, Summer, Supplement ix.

Nocon J J (2000) Shoulder Dystocia and Macrosomia. In L H Kean, P N Baker, and D I Edelstone, *Best Practice in Labor Ward Management.* Harcourt: London.

Olugbile A and Mascarenhas L (2000) Review of Shoulder Dystocia at the Birmingham Women's Hospital, *Journal of Obstetrics & Gynaecology* **20** (3), 267–70.

Resnik R (1980) Management of Shoulder Dystocia Girdle, *Clinical Obstetrics and Gynaecology* **23** (2), 559–64.

Rouse D J, Owen J, Goldenberg R L and Cliver S P (1996) The Effectiveness and Costs of Elective Cesarean Delivery for Fetal Macrosomia Diagnosed by Ultrasound, *Journal of American Medical Association* **276** (18), 1480–6.

Rubin A (1964) Management of Shoulder Dystocia, *Journal of American Medical Association* **189**, 835–7.

Sama J C and Iffy L (1998) Maternal Weight and Fetal Injury at Birth: Data Arising From Medico-Legal Research, *Medicine and Law* **17** (1), 61–8.

Smeltzer J S (1986) Prevention and Management of Shoulder Dystocia, *Clinical Obstetrics and Gynaecology* **29** (2), 299–308.

Spellacy W N, Miller S, Winegar A and Peterson P Q (1985) Macrosomia – Maternal Characteristics and Infant Complications, *Obstetrics Gynaecology* **66**, 158–160.

Spong C Y, Beall M and Rodrigues D (1995) An Objective Definition of Shoulder Dystocia: Prolonged Head to Body Delivery Intervals and/or the Use of Ancillary Obstetric Manoeuvres, *Obstetrics and Gynaecology* **86**, 433–6.

Stirrat G M and Taylor R W (2002) Mechanisms of Obstetric Brachial Plexus Palsy: A Critical Analysis, *Clinical Risk* **8**, 218–22.

Swartz B C and Dixon D M (1958) Shoulder Dystocia, *Obstetrics and Gynaecology* **11**, 468–71.

Toohey J S, Keegan K A., Morgan M A, Francis J, Task S and deVenciana M (1995) The 'Dangerous Multipara': Fact or Fiction?, *American Journal of Obstetrics and Gynaecology* **172**, 683–6.

Woods C E (1943) A Principle of Physics as Applied to Shoulder Dystocia, *American Journal of Obstetrics and Gynaecology* **45**, 796–805.

5

The Birth of Undiagnosed Twins in the Community

Pat Lindsay

Introduction

Until recently multiple pregnancy was a relatively uncommon event, occurring in approximately one in eighty births. The last twenty years have seen an increase in twin births, which now have an incidence of one in forty-three pregnancies (Smith-Levitin et al. 1999). This is partly explained by the development of assisted reproductive technology. The trend towards delayed and later childbearing has also had an impact, as older women have a higher incidence of naturally occurring multiple pregnancies. Ethnic variations also occur: in some Nigerian communities the incidence of twins is as high as between one in twenty and one in twenty-five (Blackburn 2003 p. 123).

Most twin pregnancies are diagnosed well before labour begins, usually on ultrasound scan in the first or second trimester, and women are advised to arrange for the birth in an obstetric consultant unit. This chapter outlines the diagnosis of multiple pregnancy in the absence of ultrasonography, when women fail to take up antenatal care, for example, and how health professionals might manage an emergency delivery of twins in the community including external cephalic version (ECV) and internal podalic version (IPV). The principles of care during the birth may also be applied to cases where a woman chooses to have a twin birth at home despite professional advice to attend hospital (see, for example, Cronk 1992).

Diagnosis of twins/multiple pregnancy during labour

Because of the routine use of ultrasound scans in pregnancy, it is very rare for twins to be diagnosed for the first time in labour. However, if a woman elects not to have an ultrasound scan, midwives should be familiar with symptoms suggestive (but not diagnostic) of multiple pregnancy. These include feelings of extreme tiredness and exaggerated minor disorders, such as morning sickness, varicosities, heartburn and backache (multiparous women may compare this pregnancy unfavourably to their previous experiences). Nonetheless, there are situations when midwives may be faced with the unexpected delivery of twins in the community. For example, very young or unsupported women may conceal their pregnancy and avoid antenatal care (even multiple pregnancies can be concealed very successfully with judicious choice of clothing). Women with bad memories of previous pregnancies and births may similarly choose to 'go it alone'. Occasionally the woman's social circumstances make it difficult for her to attend, such as is the case with travelling families or those who are illegal residents.

The presence of even one of the following clinical findings should alert the midwife to the possibility of twins:

- fundal height higher than expected for the period of gestation;
- abdominal girth greater than 100 cm in an average-sized woman (Hofmeyr and Drakeley 1998);
- lateral borders of the uterus extend out into the flanks and contain fetal parts;
- at least three fetal poles palpable (that is, two heads and one breech or two breeches and one head);
- multiple fetal limbs palpable;
- fetal hearts loud and clearly heard in two different uterine quadrants, with rates differing by at least ten beats (and neither of them synchronous with the maternal pulse);
- birth of a baby much smaller than anticipated and uterus which remains large.

First-time diagnosis of multiple pregnancy in advanced labour in the home or a woman with a multiple pregnancy choosing home birth presents risks for mother and fetuses and, in order to detect any risk to the health of the mother and/or fetuses/babies at the earliest moment, it is important to be aware of the potential complications of twin delivery. The potential hazards need to be discussed with the woman and her partner. If all parties clearly understand the risks and actions which are necessary to maximise safety, they are more likely to be co-operative. A relationship of mutual trust is essential.

Potential complications

Fetal/neonatal complications

Complications and aberrations of development present a risk for twin fetuses. Perinatal mortality is up to six times higher than for a singleton pregnancy and monochorionic twins are at particular risk (Neilson and Bajoria 2001, Blackburn 2003, p. 122). Placental abnormalities are commoner and include vascular anastamoses, velamentous cord insertion and vasa praevia. This increases the likelihood of serious haematological problems both before and after birth. Developmental abnormalities occur more frequently and include chromosomal anomalies, gastro-intestinal atresias, cardiac defects, cerebral lesions, conjoined twins, and acardiac fetus. Cord entanglement may occur in monoamnionic twins and this may lead to the death of one or both twins. Growth restriction is common, either as a result of twin-to-twin-transfusion syndrome or poor transplacental transfer of nutrients (Neilson and Bajoria 2001), and preterm birth is a risk for either monozygotic or dizygotic twins. Polyhydramnios is commoner than in singleton pregnancies and this may favour non-engagement of the first twin, unstable lie and the risk of cord prolapse when the membranes rupture. There is a higher incidence of cerebral palsy, particularly in monozygotic twins (Neilson and Bajoria 2001). During the birth the risk of fetal hypoxia is increased for both infants, but more especially so for the second twin.

Maternal complications

Multiple pregnancy is riskier for the mother. Pre-eclampsia is more of a risk than for a singleton pregnancy and anaemia may also be a problem, owing to the heavier fetal demand for iron. There is an increased incidence of obstetric cholestasis and acute fatty liver of pregnancy and antepartum haemorrhage occurs more frequently in twin pregnancies, the majority being placental abruption (Smith-Levitin et al. 1999). Intrapartum haemorrhage due to separation of the placenta of the first twin is a unique hazard in multiple births.

After delivery, the uterus, overdistended in pregnancy, may not maintain contraction, and atonic postpartum haemorrhage is more likely. The effects of any haemorrhage will be made worse if the woman is also anaemic (Crowther 1999). The Report *Why Mothers Die 1997–1999* (NICE 2001) indicates a maternal mortality rate of 20.1 per 100,000 twin maternities (21.5 per 100,000 triplet maternities), compared with a maternal mortality rate of 11.2 for singletons. In addition, there are the potential psychological, social and financial consequences of giving birth to unexpected twins.

Management

The following account of the management of a twin birth at home addresses the scenario that a midwife receives an emergency call and arrives at the woman's home and labour is advanced.

Assess and discuss findings (Figure 5.1)

On arrival at the woman's home, the midwife must make a rapid assessment of the situation. The midwife will make a thorough clinical examination and take a history of the pregnancy and labour.

Assessment will include measurement of temperature, pulse respirations (as time permits) and blood pressure, abdominal examination and auscultation of the fetal hearts. It is essential that the midwife ascertains the presentation and lie of the fetuses. At this stage it is unwise to assume that only two infants are present – undiagnosed triplets are not unknown. The state of the membranes, colour of the liquor (if ruptured) and uterine activity is assessed. Following her/his assessment, the midwife must make a decision about care management and discuss it with the woman. In the situation that the woman is clearly in advanced labour and the clinical signs indicate that this is an undiagnosed multiple pregnancy, the woman (and her partner) must be made aware of the midwife's suspicion of twin pregnancy and the likelihood that there will not be time to transfer to hospital.

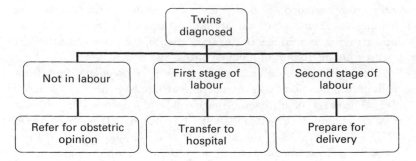

Figure 5.1   Summary of assessment and decision-making on first diagnosis of twin pregnancy

Call for assistance (Figure 5.2)

The midwife must call for emergency medical assistance (Rule 40, UKCC 1998). The local consultant maternity unit should be informed and the assistance of another two midwives requested. A paramedic ambulance, with obstetric and neonatal facilities, should be called.

Prepare for the birth (Figure 5.2)

While waiting for help to arrive, the midwife must make arrangements for the birth. A calm, unflustered atmosphere is essential to avoid panic and to reassure the woman that she is able to birth her babies herself with the help of the midwife. The birth should take place in a warm, private area, with adequate lighting and enough room for the midwife and the woman to work together. The partner can be asked to find the following equipment:

- clean towels for the babies
- clean and warm cot
- extra set of baby clothes
- clean linen (including sheets and towels) for the birth area
- clean towel for the midwife (for hand hygiene).

If the midwife has specific equipment, for example a delivery pack, extra cord clamps, gloves, infant resuscitation equipment and

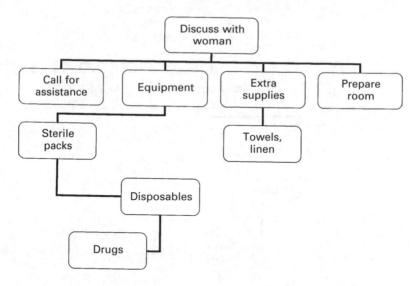

Figure 5.2 Summary of preparations for the birth

Entonox®, these can be brought into the room. If this is an unplanned emergency twin birth, especially in the absence of any antenatal care, the midwife can insert a size 16-gauge intravenous cannula *if time permits*. Collection of blood for 'group and save serum' now might also be useful should there be a need for cross-matching later.

Assist with the birth (Figure 5.3)

The midwife must monitor maternal and fetal wellbeing and make clear records of the decisions made, the actions taken, the care given and the results of maternal and fetal observations (Rule 42, UKCC 1998). The time of all events should be recorded, as is usual during a birth.

A vaginal examination should be made when the membranes rupture, to exclude cord prolapse and confirm presentation, position and descent. This is especially important if the first twin appears to be a breech presentation. The woman should be asked to empty her bladder. Water may be given to drink if she wishes but food is inadvisable at this stage in a complicated birth.

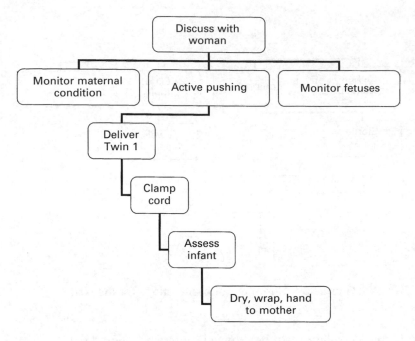

Figure 5.3   Summary of the birth of twin one

When active pushing begins, the woman should be helped to find a comfortable birth position. Upright positions are useful as they maximise the space in the pelvic outlet and allow the normal mechanism of labour to proceed unhindered (Russell 1982). They also help fetal oxygenation by avoiding supine hypotensive syndrome, which may occur when recumbent positions are used (Blackburn 2003 p. 266). There is no need for interventions such as episiotomy unless there is a clear indication, for example fetal bradycardia in late second stage.

When the first baby is born, the midwife will note the time, assess its condition, dry it and wrap it in dry towels in order to prevent hypothermia. The woman can be encouraged to hold her baby. Two clamps should be used to divide the umbilical cord; it is essential that the placental end of the cord is not allowed to drain as this risks exsanguination of the second twin should this be a monochorionic gestation. If this happens, the midwife can expect the second twin to be in very poor condition at birth. The first baby should clearly identified as 'twin one'.

This is to avoid confusion for the midwife and the woman if both babies are the same sex.

The midwife must now assess the condition, presentation and lie of the second twin by abdominal examination, followed by vaginal examination if necessary (Figure 5.4). It is usual for the contractions to cease for a few minutes at this point, which gives the midwife time to make an assessment of the second fetus. Very often the lie is longitudinal and the presenting part is in or entering the pelvic brim. In this case the midwife can encourage the woman to move to an upright position. With the aid of gravity the presenting part will start to descend and contractions will recommence. The condition of the second twin must be monitored. If all

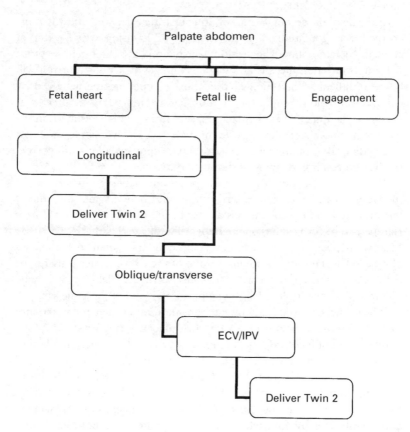

Figure 5.4   Summary of the birth of twin two

is well, the midwife can await events; there is little evidence that a prolonged time interval after the birth of the first twin has a detrimental effect on the wellbeing of the second (Barrett and Ritchie 2002). The midwife may consider rupturing the membranes (with the woman's consent) when the presenting part is in the pelvic cavity (at the level of the ischial spines) and the woman is actively pushing. However, artificial rupture of the membranes commits the midwife to completing the delivery as soon as possible and removes the option of 'wait and see'. It is unwise to make such an irrevocable manoeuvre unless the midwife is certain that delivery can be achieved and potential complications (such as cord presentation) have been excluded. All clinical decisions should be discussed with the woman and documented, including decisions to 'wait and see' (UKCC 1998).

If the lie of the second twin is oblique or transverse, the midwife must correct it to longitudinal as soon as possible using either external cephalic or internal podalic version as explained in subsequent sections. It is important that there is no delay, as once contractions return it will be very difficult. Correction of the lie can sometimes be achieved by external cephalic version if the membranes are intact. As an attempt at version in labour may cause placental separation with a resultant intra-partum haemorrhage, the midwife must observe the woman for any sign of bleeding. Internal podalic version may be required. This will correct the lie and result in delivery of the second twin as a breech.

When the presenting part is in the pelvis and active pushing resumes, the woman can be assisted to birth the second baby. Again, the time of birth is noted and the condition is assessed. The umbilical cord is securely clamped. Two cord clamps on the baby will indicate that this is 'twin two'. Most women very quickly learn to recognise the individual characteristics of their twins. However, some indication of their birth order is useful for the midwife, who has to record details such as birth-weight for each baby and may find it difficult to tell them apart if they are of the same sex.

The midwife must now palpate the woman's abdomen and make sure that the uterus is empty of all but the placenta (Figure 5.5). Active management of the third stage of labour is advisable, as there is a higher risk of postpartum haemorrhage due to atonic uterus, as mentioned earlier (Neilson and Bajoria 2001). If an oxytocic drug is available, it can with the woman's consent, be given, once the midwife is sure that no third fetus is in the uterus. This is followed by delivery of the placentae and membranes by controlled cord traction, grasping both cords and applying traction to both simultaneously.

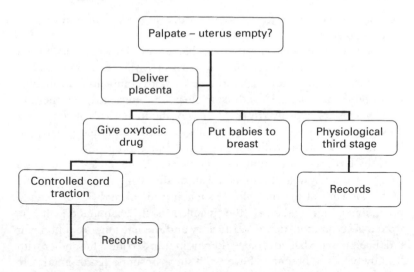

Figure 5.5 Summary of the third stage of labour

If no oxytocic drug is available, the woman can be encouraged to suckle the babies while the midwife awaits the expulsion of the placenta and membranes. Physiological management of the third stage has been discussed (Evans 1997). However, it should not be undertaken unless the midwife is sure that these are dizygotic twins. The woman must give her informed consent.

The placentae and membranes must be examined carefully and disposed of in accordance with local policy. In some areas placentae from multiple gestations are sent for histological examination to determine zygosity.

In the absence of information about maternal blood type, the midwife (after discussion and obtaining consent) should take blood samples from both placentae for fetal blood typing and a direct Coombs test, and from the mother for a Kleihauer test. The genital tract should be inspected for trauma and any suturing required should be undertaken. The woman's condition should be reassessed and her personal hygiene attended to. She will then need time to rest quietly with her partner and the babies. This is a good opportunity for the midwife to complete the records. Detailed records are essential and should include all decisions made, all care given, the time of calling for skilled assistance, and the time that help arrived. When the events are over, the midwife should report the incident to her supervisor of midwives as soon as possible.

It is important to ensure that the babies are fed early and do not become cold. Twins are commonly born at earlier gestations and at lower birth-weights than singleton infants. With competition for maternal resources in pregnancy and relatively poorer nutrient stores, they are at higher risk of hypoglycæmia. In view of the higher risk of congenital anomaly, the babies should be carefully examined and their progress in the first hours and days after birth carefully monitored.

If the birth was at term and straightforward, the babies are of good weight and all is well, the mother can, if she wishes, remain at home under the care of the midwife. A suitably trained midwife or general practitioner can undertake the detailed birth examination. If the woman's accommodation is satisfactory and she has support at home, it is difficult to see what advantage there is in transferring a fit mother with healthy babies to hospital. However, if she is unsupported or in adverse social circumstances, transfer to hospital may be in her best interests. Similarly, if complications arose during the birth, or the condition of the mother or either of the babies gives cause for concern, they must be admitted without delay.

Postnatal care of the mother must include careful observation of her reaction to and management of her babies. Emotional reactions following this unexpected and possibly traumatic event may occur. If any invasive manoeuvre, such as internal podalic version, has been used, antibiotics should be prescribed and the woman must be watched for signs of endometritis.

The midwife should make sure that the woman has information about benefits available and the contact details if there is a local twins club (TAMBA (Twins and Multiple Birth Association) or similar). The parents will be facing unexpected emotional and financial challenges and will probably welcome this information.

External cephalic version

External cephalic version (ECV) may be attempted in an effort to convert a transverse or oblique lie to longitudinal. The aim is to achieve a cephalic fetal presentation. The procedure carries a risk of trauma and haemorrhage for the mother and feto-maternal haemorrhage, cord entanglement and hypoxia for the fetus, especially during labour (Penn

1999). ECV is also not always successful and may lead to further complications such as compound presentation, cord prolapse and fetal hypoxia (Novak-Antolič 1998). In an undiagnosed twin birth, therefore, the midwife would not use it to convert a breech to a cephalic presentation as in this situation a controlled breech delivery is the safer option. However, oblique or transverse lie cannot be left uncorrected as both will result in obstructed labour.

The woman will need to lie on her back, with a slight lateral tilt, while the midwife assesses the lie, the presentation and the heart rate of the second twin. With one hand on the maternal abdomen against the fetal head and the other against the breech, the midwife gently pushes the head towards the maternal pelvis (Figure 5.6). When the head is above

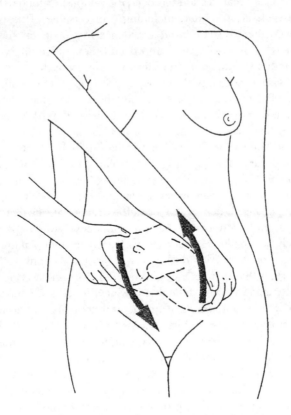

Figure 5.6 External cephalic version

the pelvis, the fetal heart should be recorded. The whole manoeuvre should not take more than ten minutes (Penn 1999). Once the fetal head is in the pelvic brim, the woman can be encouraged to adopt an upright position to facilitate descent.

The chances of successful external version are slim if the uterus is contracting or the membranes of the second sac are ruptured. An attempt at external version in these circumstances carries a high risk of maternal and fetal trauma. If external version fails to correct an oblique or transverse lie, the midwife must attempt an internal podalic version.

Internal podalic version

Until recently Caesarean section has been the established mode of delivery for transverse lie in labour, including transverse lie of the second twin. However, there is some limited evidence that neonatal and long-term outcomes are not necessarily improved by operative intervention, and evidence that Caesarean section for the delivery of the second twin increases maternal morbidity (Drew et al. 1991, Chauhan et al. 2001, Crowther 2002). The art of internal podalic version has, therefore, recently seen a revival (Figure 5.7). The midwife may need to carry out an internal podalic version during the birth if the lie of the second twin is found to be oblique or transverse. In this situation labour becomes obstructed and there is a real danger of prolapse of the cord or a fetal arm once the membranes rupture. Fetal damage or death is then likely. Internal podalic version will correct the lie and expedite delivery of the fetus by assisted breech delivery or breech extraction (Crowther 1999). Drew et al. in 1991 considered that this manoeuvre was required for approximately one in fifteen second twins. For an account of a midwife's use of internal podalic version during a twin birth, see Cronk 1992.

It is important that there is the minimum of delay in carrying it out, as successful version is very difficult to achieve once the contractions have returned. Some authorities recommend that an attempt at internal podalic version is made before the membranes rupture. If the membranes are intact, the presence of the liquor will assist the manoeuvre by increasing fetal mobility and minimising uterine moulding around the fetus (Rabinovici et al. 1988, Novak-Antolič 1998, Hofmeyr & Drakeley 1998). If the membranes are ruptured, the manoeuvre must be carried out at once, before too much liquor has drained away.

The situation must be explained to the woman and her consent

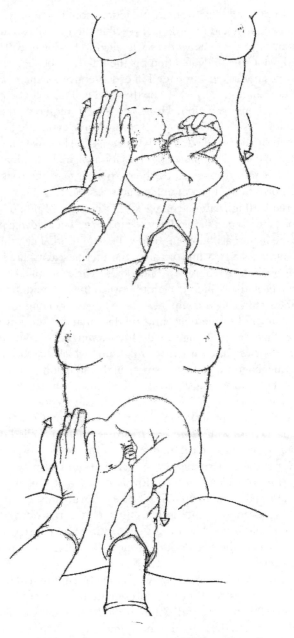

Figure 5.7 Internal podalic version

obtained to proceed. The woman's bladder should be empty. The fetal heart is auscultated and recorded. If possible the midwife should put on a clean pair of gloves. The woman will need to lie down, with her back supported, while the midwife attempts the internal podalic version. The lithotomy position is recommended in order to give adequate access and facilitate descent and delivery (Crowther 1999). This may be difficult to achieve in a home situation. However, if it is required, the position described for version during home birth by Berkeley in 1922 may work. The woman should be asked to lie down across the bed, with her buttocks at the edge of the bed and knees bent (as for a vaginal examination). The legs and feet can be supported by the partner or over the back of chairs beside the bed. Some form of analgesia is desirable as this procedure is uncomfortable. If inhalational analgesia (for example, Entonox, ® BOC) is available, the woman should be asked to use it. The midwife places one hand on the maternal abdomen, below the fetal head. The other hand is inserted into the vagina and up into the uterine cavity until a foot is located through the membranes. The foot is clearly identified by the presence of the heel, the right angle joint between the foot and the lower leg, the shortness of the digits compared to the fingers on hand, the length of the sole compared to the palm and the fact that toes do not grasp the examining finger as fetal fingers will. It is **essential** that the midwife is sure that it is ***the foot and not the hand*** which has been grasped. Traction on a hand would be disastrous in this situation and would cause transverse lie with prolapse of the fetal arm. Labour will become obstructed and the only option then is Caesarean section.

On locating the foot, it should be firmly grasped between the first and second fingers and, with ***slow continuous*** traction, pulled down into the vagina, while the external hand assists the version by pushing the head towards the upper pole of the uterus. (Both feet may be brought down together provided that the midwife is sure that s(he) has not inadvertently grasped a hand and a foot.) The midwife must ensure that the fetal back is guided to lie anteriorly as the foot is drawn down. Failure to do so may result in the descent of the fetus in a sacroposterior position and entrapment of the fetal occiput in the hollow of the maternal sacrum during delivery.

If the membranes are intact, they can then be ruptured and the infant delivered as an assisted breech presentation or breech extraction (Crowther 1999, Barrett and Ritchie 2002). Internal podalic version carries risks for both the fetus and the woman. Fetal hypoxia is likely and the midwife should be prepared to resuscitate the infant. Fetal trauma is sometimes associated with assisted breech delivery. This includes fractures of the long bones. Maternal trauma, such as shock due to pain, rupture of the uterus, and vaginal wall damage can occur, so the procedure should not be carried out forcefully. As it is so invasive, endometritis and puerperal infection is a possibility.

Any attempt at either external or internal version must only be done with the informed consent of the woman.

Supervisor of midwives' commentary

With modern technology it is generally expected that a multiple pregnancy will be identified, but, as the chapter suggests, some women will elect not to have an ultrasound scan, and the undiagnosed twins scenario can occur. Whilst scanning can be regarded as a very useful diagnostic tool, I am aware that fairly recently a mother gave birth to twins which had not been diagnosed at her routine scans.

The chapter reminds us of the exaggerated minor disorders of pregnancy that these mothers may experience and the potential clinical indicators which, if identified, would alert the midwife to suspect a multiple pregnancy, but this is not always the case and a midwife could find herself in a situation similar to the scenario at the end of this chapter.

Unplanned home births can cause a degree of excitement but to attend a labouring mother at home and discover a twin pregnancy requires utmost competence and confidence. In such a situation not only will the mother require much physical and emotional support but so will her partner and family.

Any community-based midwife must, therefore, make sure her skills remain up to date. If she works in a patch where very few home births occur, she should ensure some rotation on to the delivery suite for normal delivery experience. If she is unable to organise this for herself then she should seek the support of her supervisor of midwives to enable this to happen. *'Supervisors of midwives will strive to ensure that midwives have a positive relationship with their supervisor that: facilitates safe and autonomous practice and promotes accountability'* (ENB 1999).

Any midwife will benefit from reading chapters such as this one, as well as attending regular training sessions which include management of emergency scenarios.

Key points

* If multiple pregnancy is suspected confirm diagnosis as soon as possible.

- Call for appropriate help.
- Ensure adequate supplies of equipment, for example cord clamps.
- Inform the supervisor of midwives and the obstetric unit of the imminent births and keep them updated of progress.
- Maintain contemporaneous notes (Rule 42, Midwives Rules and Code of Practice UKCC 1998), including not only fetal heart rates, times of delivery, Apgar scores, etc., but also any manoeuvres required to assist delivery, for example during breech delivery.
- Before administering an oxytocic drug, palpate the uterus to exclude the presence of another fetus.

Obstetric commentary

Twin gestations frequently involve maternal and fetal complications, and are quite often considered as 'premium' pregnancies. Having two fetuses in the uterus increases the risks to both mother and babies. Twin pregnancies are prone to a virtual doubling of all risks for complications when compared to a singleton pregnancy. The overall perinatal mortality is ten times higher than in singletons (dichorionic 9 per cent, monochorionic 26 per cent, monoamniotic 50 per cent). The increased morbidity and mortality is due to prematurity (50 per cent of twins weigh less than 2500 g), Intrauterine growth retardation (30–50 per cent), and congenital abnormalities (twice as high). Pre-eclampsia occurs in about 10 to 20 per cent of women carrying twins, twice the rate of women pregnant with one baby.

The optimal mode of delivery of twin pregnancy remains controversial, in particular if the presentation is not vertex–vertex. Forty per cent of twins present as vertex–vertex. However, even in these cases the second twin may become non-vertex after the delivery of the first twin. When the first baby is a vertex presentation, vaginal delivery is recommended. A non-vertex presentation of the first twin is generally considered as an indication for Caesarean section, mainly owing to lack of evidence about the safety of vaginal delivery.

The second twin should be monitored continuously after the delivery of the first twin. Determine the lie and position of the second twin and wait for the presenting part to descend into the pelvis and be at the spines or below before rupturing the membranes. If the second twin is non-cephalic, version may be attempted. Use external cephalic version with intact membranes only and internal podalic version and breech extraction with ruptured membranes.

Limiting the time interval between the two babies to 30 minutes has been advocated to reduce the risks of placental abruption, cord prolapse and birth asphyxia to the second twin. Several reports have shown no correlation between five minutes Apgar scores and the interval between the twins. It is recommended that if labour is not established after the delivery of the first baby, amniotomy should be considered when the presenting part is in the pelvis.

Second twins born at term are at higher risk of death due to complications during labour and delivery than first twins. The mortality rate of second twins born at term is approximately 1 in 270 (mainly due to intrapartum anoxia, most cases of which result from mechanical problems after vaginal delivery of first twins). Since the excess of deaths of second twins at term seems to be attributable to labour, current data suggest that planned Caesarean delivery may be protective against perinatal death among twins. Women with twins should be counselled about the risk to the second twin and the theoretical possibility of a protective effect of planned Caesarean section. About 15 per cent of second twins are delivered by Caesarean section after vaginal delivery of the first twin.

The average blood loss in the vaginal delivery of twins is 500 ml greater than for a singleton. This is likely to be due to a large placental bed as well as uterine overdistension leading to atony. Active management of the third stage is therefore advocated.

Home delivery of twins is considered by most obstetricians as a less than ideal setting because of the lack of provision of:

- continuous and simultaneous fetal monitoring of fetal hearts;
- ultrasound that may be required to assess the second twin presentation;
- appropriate analgesia and/or anaesthesia if internal manipulation is required, for example internal podalic version and breech extraction or immediate delivery by Caesarean section;
- an experienced attendant familiar with external cephalic version, vaginal breech delivery, as well as breech extraction if required;
- advanced neonatal resuscitation.

Key points

- The incidence of multiple pregnancies is increasing owing to infertility treatments.
- Twins should be considered as a high-risk pregnancy and birth.
- Home delivery of twins may not be appropriate because of the lack of facilities.
- If practical and acceptable to the mother, transfer from the community into the hospital.
- Vaginal delivery is the preferred mode of delivery if the first twin is presenting with the vertex (70 per cent of cases).

- Caesarean section should be considered when the first twin is a non-vertex presentation and in monoamniotic twins.

A problem-based scenario and interactive action planning exercise
The birth of undiagnosed twins in the community

Rose lives in a rural village approximately forty miles from the nearest maternity unit. She is 38 years old and a gravida 9, para 8, and is pregnant again. She is a slim woman, weighing 52 kg.

You are visiting her to carry out the booking interview. During the course of your discussion you learn the following information:

- All previous babies were normal deliveries, with no complications. The most recent labour lasted one hour.
- Rose is healthy with no history of illness or operations.
- Her aunts on her mother's side are twins.
- Rose is feeling very tired and is more than usually sick this time.
- Last menstrual period dates suggest a gestation period of 15 weeks. Rose has felt movements for the last 2 weeks.

What are the risk factors in Rose's personal history which make her higher risk for twins?

What aspects of her current condition suggest that this pregnancy is different?

Are there any other conditions which might produce similar symptoms (differential diagnosis)?

You have probably identified the following risk factors:

- Older mother.
- Multiparous.
- Maternal family history of twinning.

Current condition

- Unusual tiredness.
- Very early fetal movements.
- Complaints of unusual vomiting in pregnancy. (*Note*: Rose is an experienced mother and recognises that this is not the usual pattern for her pregnancies.)

→

Differential diagnosis

- Wrong dates.
- Hydatidiform mole.

Write down what action is necessary.

Your plan of care should include the following:

- Explore the accuracy of the menstrual dates.
- Make an appointment for a scan as soon as possible.
- Arrange a follow-up antenatal visit after the scan result.

Rose fails to attend for her scan appointment and for her next antenatal visit. On investigation you learn that she has left the area.

Approximately 24 weeks after your meeting with Rose you are on call for the community at night. You receive a telephone call at 11 p.m. It is Rose's partner. They have recently moved back to the area and Rose is now 39 weeks pregnant (she is sure of her dates). She is having frequent contractions and is refusing to go in to hospital. He asks you to attend at once.

What do you do?

Your action plan should include:

- The house address and directions for you.
- Brief information about Rose's state of health and health of the pregnancy.
- Following local protocol to inform another team member of your whereabouts.
- Collection of equipment for a home birth.

Owing to sickness there is no other team member available to cover you or come to assist. Rose's partner tells you that she has had no antenatal care since she last saw you. The hand-held notes you started were lost some months ago.

Taking your equipment and drugs, you set out to attend the call. On arrival at the house, Rose is obviously in advanced labour. After assessing her condition you palpate the uterus. These are your findings:

- The uterine fundus reaches the xyphisternum.
- Fetal parts are felt in flanks and in midline.
- Three fetal poles are identified (two heads, one breech), one head is in the fundus, the other is in the pelvic brim.
- A fetal heart is heard in the right lower quadrant: 130 beats per minute.
- A fetal heart is heard in the right upper quadrant: 144 beats per minute (Rose's pulse is 96 beats per minute).
- Rose is having strong contractions, three to four contractions every ten minutes and lasting 50 seconds.

What is your assessment of the situation?

What is your plan of care now?

Your answer should include the following:

- The clinical findings are strongly suggestive of multiple pregnancy.
- This may be twins; it may be triplets – you cannot be sure at this stage.
- Multiple birth is hazardous for both mother and babies, and is better conducted in hospital.
- Urgent transfer to hospital is in the best interests of mother and babies, especially as Rose has had no antenatal care.
- You will discuss this with Rose and her partner and emphasise the need for transfer.

As you are telling Rose your findings, the membranes rupture and Rose begins to push.

What are you going to do now?

Your actions should include the following:

- Call at once for urgent assistance from the paramedic ambulance service.
- Alert the maternity unit that you are dealing with the delivery of undiagnosed twins at home, who might require neonatal care.
- Insert a size 16-gauge intravenous cannula if there is time. Take blood if there is time.
- Ask the partner to collect clean linen to cover the birth area.
- Assist Rose into a comfortable position.
- Open the equipment you have brought with you and prepare for the birth.
- Deliver Twin 1.
- Clamp the cord twice and divide between the clamps.
- Hand the baby to Rose and dry it well to prevent heat loss.
- Ask Rose to lie down and palpate the lie of the second twin.
- Correct the lie if it is not longitudinal, rupture the membranes when it is safe to do so and deliver the baby.
- Await the return of contractions if the lie is longitudinal.
- Deliver the baby.
- Palpate the uterus to exclude the presence of another fetus.
- Active management of the third stage of labour.
- Make a careful assessment of uterine contraction and retraction.
- Make a careful assessment of blood loss.
- Consider collecting blood samples from the placentae and from the mother.

References

Barrett J F R and Ritchie W K (2002) Twin Delivery, *Best Practice and Research in Clinical Obstetrics and Gynaecology* **16** (1), 43–56.

Chauhan A R, Singhal T T and Raut V S (2001) Is Internal Podalic Version a Lost Art? Optimum Mode of Delivery in Transverse Lie, *Journal of Postgraduate Medicine* **47**, 15–8.

Cronk M (1992) A Doubly Difficult Birth, *Nursing Times* **88** (47) 54–6.

Crowther C A (1999) Multiple Pregnancy. In D K James, P J Steer, C P Weiner and B Gonik, *High Risk Pregnancy, Management Options* (2nd edn). Saunders: London.

Crowther C A (2002) Caesarean Delivery for the Second Twin (Cochrane Review). In *The Cochrane Library*, Issue 4, 2002, Oxford: Update Software.

Drew J H, McKenzie J, Kelly E and Beischer N (1991) Second Twin: Quality of Survival if Born by Breech Extraction Following Internal Podalic Version *Australian New Zealand Journal of Obstetrics and Gynaecology* **31** (2), 111–4.

ENB (1999) *Advice and Guidance for Local Supervising Authorities and Supervisor of Midwives*. English National Board for Nursing, Midwifery and Health Visiting: London.

Evans J (1997) Can a Twin Birth be a Positive Experience?, *Midwifery Matters*, **Issue 74**, Autumn, 6–11.

Hofmeyr G F and Drakeley A J (1998) Delivery of Twins, *Baillière's Clinical Obstetrics and Gynaecology* **12** (1), 91–107.

Neilson J P and Bajoria R (2001) Multiple Pregnancy. In G Chamberlain and P Steer, *Turnbull's Obstetrics* (3rd edn). Churchill Livingstone: London.

NICE (National Institute for Clinical Excellence) (2001) *Why Mothers Die 1997–1999; The Confidential Enquiries into Maternal Deaths in the United Kingdom*. Royal College Obstetricians and Gynaecology Press: London.

Novak-Antolič Ž (1998) Abnormal Presentations: Transverse Lie, Brow and Face Presentations. In A Kurjak (Editor in Chief), *Textbook of Perinatal Medicine*. Parthenon Publishing Group: London.

Penn Z (1999) Breech Presentation. In D James, P Steer, C Weiner and B Gonik, (eds) *High Risk Pregnancy, Management Options*. Saunders: London.

Rabinovici J, Barkai G, Reichman B, Serr D M and Mashiach S (1988) Internal Podalic Version With Unruptured Membranes For The Second Twin in Transverse Lie, *Obstetrics and Gynecology* **73** (3), Part 1, 428–30.

Russell J G B (1982) The Rationale of Primitive Delivery Positions *British Journal of Obstetrics and Gynaecology* **89**, 712–5.

Smith-Levitin M, Skupski D W and Chervenak F A (1999) Multifetal Pregnancies: Epidemiology, Clinical Characteristics and Management. In E A Reece and J C Hobbins, *Medicine of the Fetus and Mother*. Lippincott-Raven: Philadelphia: PA.

UKCC (United Kingdom Central Council for Nursing, Midwifery and Health Visiting) (1998) *Midwives Rules and Code of Practice*. UKCC: London.

6

Managing Breech Presentation in the Absence of Obstetric Assistance

Susan Burvill

Introduction

Although the fear culture in the West surrounding breech births may have given it 'emergency' status, for many birth attendants in the world community breech birth is part of normal practice, as it was in Britain not so long ago (Allison 1996). Recently I was doing some work in a former Soviet Union country with community midwives when one day a midwife arrived late for a seminar. She calmly said, 'Sorry I am late. I just had a woman arrive at the clinic and give birth to twins, both breech!' In fact, my own first breech experience was in Africa with a midwife who commented that the occasional breech in the day made midwifery interesting. I do not dispute the raised perinatal mortality and morbidity rates of breech babies, but I would contend that the perception of vaginal breech birth as an 'emergency' reflects the lack of experience. It is this lack of experience that engenders fear, which in turn impedes both midwifery skill learning and women's options.

Based on the view that it is of paramount importance to maintain choices in childbirth, and concern that Caesarean section is becoming the norm for breech delivery, this chapter sets out principles of care and action during a physiological vaginal breech birth. This aims to support maternal choice and provide guidance for safe and confident care when

111

a breech presentation is diagnosed unexpectedly during advanced labour in a community setting.

Breech presentation at term: the issue of choice and vaginal breech birth

The opportunity for choice and the ability to be involved in and influence the decisions that affect our lives is important to individuals and fundamental to good midwifery practice in supporting women. Choice is a hallmark of good practice within the New NHS and 'informed choice' is an essential requirement in the provision of professional practice (DoH 1993, DoH 2000a).

Based on my practice as an independent midwife, women and their partners are increasingly raising questions about and rejecting practices and procedures which are not evidence-based but merely 'traditional' modes of care. The choice about how their baby should be born must always remain with the parents. It is important to ensure that parents are not coerced into informed compliance with local policy dictates (Stapleton et al. 2002, Lowdon 1998). It is essential, therefore, that they are well-informed and encouraged to choose from the options available to them. Open discussion is imperative as written information alone is not sufficient to facilitate informed choice (O'Cathain et al. 2002).

When women discover that they have a breech-presenting baby at term, ensure if possible that they are provided with choices before labour starts. For example, postural advice and alternative therapies such as moxibustion can be explored (Hawkey 1997, Hofmeyr 1996, Midwifery Today 1996). Although these methods have appeared successful only anecdotally and there is insufficient research evidence to recommend them, they can serve to empower a woman who is already in a vulnerable situation. Obstetric procedures such as external cephalic version (ECV) (Hofmeyr 2004), medical-led breech vaginal delivery and Caesarean section (RCOG 1999), as well as the availability of skills for vaginal breech birth in the area where you work, should be discussed so that women can make an informed decision.

The 'Term Breech Trial' (Hannah el al. 2000) was an international, multicentre, randomised controlled trial comparing vaginal breech delivery with planned Caesarean section for breech. Even so, the trial only compared medical-led vaginal deliveries with planned Caesarean sections and did not, therefore, provide information about physiological vaginal breech birth. The primary findings were that breech-presenting babies at term delivered by Caesarean section were three times less likely to die or suffer serious morbidity than medical-led breech vaginal deliveries (1.6 per cent versus 5 per cent). The study's conclusion that Caesarean section provides the safest option for breech presentation was quickly disseminated, and it is anticipated that women's choice may be restricted as a consequence (Banks 2002). With diminishing skill in vaginal breech birth which may result, it is only a matter of time before women will find it difficult to find health professionals to support their wishes for a vaginal breech birth (Thornton and Hayman 2002, Robinson 2000, Robson et al. 1999, Hannah and Hannah 1996).

However, critics have suggested that the Hannah study has a number of methodological weaknesses which bring into the question the extent to which the findings should contribute to the evidence supporting Caesarean section as the optimum mode of delivery for breech presentation at term (Roosmalen and Rosendaal 2002, Keirse 2002). One concern is that the trial was stopped early and was therefore unable to estimate long-term maternal morbidity associated with surgical deliveries beyond six weeks postnatally. There were problems recruiting skilled and experienced clinicians to undertake vaginal breech deliveries which will necessarily affect the outcome (Term Breech Trial Newsletter, June 2000). Care between the two study groups was not comparable. Whereas fewer than four out of five planned vaginal breeches had an obstetrician present, in all but one of the Caesarean sections this was the case. It could be argued, therefore, that the planned Caesarean section group had more attentive care. Despite these limitations, the study is likely to be extremely influential in establishing the management of breech presentation at term. As Caesarean section becomes the norm, replication will not be feasible in the UK and the future of vaginal breech birth appears destined to decline.

The implications of a policy of mandatory Caesarean section for all breech-presenting babies are far-reaching. As vaginal breech birth becomes considered beyond the sphere of normal practice, fear amongst health care professionals may increase. However, it remains essential that health professionals be prepared to provide safe, effective and confident care when required. Approximately 25 per cent of breech presentations are diagnosed during labour (Nwosu et al. 1993) when birth is imminent and Caesarean section not feasible. Interestingly, within the

Hannah Trial (Hannah et al. 2000), 9.6 per cent of those allocated to the Caesarean section group gave birth vaginally, 59 per cent as a result of diagnosis in advanced labour. Also, anecdotal evidence from consumer groups and midwives around the world suggests that women, after considering the Hannah trial, will continue to plan for a vaginal breech birth. Registered midwives in the UK are required to 'conduct spontaneous deliveries including . . . in urgent cases a breech delivery' (UKCC 1998 p. 26).

The Confidential Enquiry into Stillbirth and Death in Infancy 7th Annual Report (CESDI 2000) recommends that the most experienced available practitioner needs to be present at a vaginal breech birth. It was highlighted that the midwife could well be the only professional around but also pointed out that the paramedic or ambulance staff are often the first to arrive at a breech birth either occurring in the home or in transit. The CESDI report recommends that all units have a guideline in place for such eventualities.

The principles and care during physiological vaginal breech birth

Readers are referred to Coates (1999) and Oxorn-Foote (1986) for a review of types, positions and causes of breech presentation. Physiological vaginal breech birth can be defined as one in which the mother births her baby in the position in which she feels most comfortable, under her own power, her uterine contractions and gravity working in harmony.

The mechanism of breech birth

An understanding of the mechanism of breech birth is vital in providing safe care and assistance.

The breech birth mechanism can be divided into three parts:

1   the buttocks and lower limbs
2   the shoulders and arms
3   the head.

The mechanism of the left sacroanterior position

The buttocks and lower limbs

The lie is longitudinal, the attitude is one of complete flexion, the position is left sacroanterior. The presenting part is the anterior (left) buttock. The bitrochanteric diameter (10 cm) enters the pelvis in the left oblique diameter of the brim and the sacrum points to the left iliopectineal eminence.

Descent takes place with increased compaction. The anterior buttock reaches the pelvic floor first and rotates forward one-eighth of a circle to lie underneath the symphysis pubis. The bitrochanteric diameter now lies in the anteroposterior diameter of the pelvic outlet. The anterior buttock escapes under the symphysis pubis, the posterior buttock sweeps the perineum and the buttocks are born by lateral flexion. The anterior buttock restitutes to the mother's right side. As descent continues, the legs are spontaneously released from the vulva.

The shoulders and arms
The shoulders enter the pelvis in left oblique diameter of the pelvis. The anterior shoulder leads, rotates one-eighth of a circle forward on the pelvic floor, and the arm and shoulder escape under the symphysis pubis. The posterior arm and shoulder are then born.

The head
The head descends into the pelvis and engages when the shoulders are at the outlet of the pelvis with the saggital suture in the transverse diameter of the pelvic brim. The occiput lies in the left anterior quadrant of the pelvis. The occiput meets the pelvic floor first and rotates one-eighth of a circle forwards. The sinciput lies in the hollow of the sacrum, and the suboccipital region (nape of the neck) impinges on the undersurface of the symphysis pubis. The body also turns so that the back is towards the mother's abdomen. The chin, face and sinciput sweep the perineum, and the head is born in a flexed attitude.

Potential complications of a vaginal breech birth

Detection and prevention of risk is imperative in all births but especially in breech presentation since fetal abnormality may be the underlying cause of the malpresentation, and the mechanics of the birth itself pose risks if not competently facilitated. Umbilical cord prolapse leading to fetal asphyxia may occur with either spontaneous or artificial rupture of the membranes (Coates 1999). The incidence of cord prolapse is increased in preterm labour (a cause of breech presentation) owing to the small presenting part, and varies depending on the type of breech. The rate in frank breech is 0.5 per cent (similar to that of vertex presentation), 5 per cent for complete breech and 15 per cent for footling and knee presentation (Barrett 1991). As the fetal head descends through the pelvis it compresses the cord against the maternal pelvis, reducing oxygen supply to the fetus. Fetal asphyxia will occur if cord compression is prolonged. Also, once the body is delivered, there may be premature separation of the placenta due to contraction and retraction of the uterus, leading to fetal hypoxia.

Because the fetal head travels rapidly through the maternal pelvis, there is no time for the gradual moulding of the skull bones which usually occurs during a vertex presentation. It is important that the vault of the fetal skull births *slowly and gently* in order to avoid rapid decompression of the fetal skull which may cause tearing of the dura mater lining the brain and major blood vessels, resulting in intracerebral haemorrhage. This is the reason why obstetricians usually apply forceps to the aftercoming fetal head, and manoeuvres described below are used to ensure controlled delivery of the head.

Damage to the baby through incorrect and excessive handling during the birth may occur and includes brachial nerve paralysis and fractures of the clavicle, femur, humerus and even the cervical spine (Confino et al. 1985). The fetal liver, kidneys and adrenal glands may be damaged if the abdominal area is roughly squeezed. To avoid trauma to the internal organs the baby should be grasped and held by the pelvic girdle and not the trunk. The baby's jaw can be dislocated if the birth attendant uses the baby's mouth to create traction for the birth instead of the cheekbones in the Mauriceau–Smellie–Veit manoeuvre.

Maternal position for breech delivery

Although upright positions in vertex presentations have been shown to have substantial benefits (Nikodem 1995), no research has been undertaken to compare the effects of maternal position on the outcomes of breech vaginal birth. In my own experience, most women spontaneously adopt a variety of positions during second stage of labour. However, it would be almost impossible to help the woman birth on her back on the floor as you would have no space to conduct any of the hands-on manoeuvres. Remember that the angle of the maternal pelvis, the expulsive contractions and the degree of gravity assist the breech to birth.

The semi-recumbent, adapted lithotomy position

In contemporary textbooks, descriptions of the manoeuvres to assist fetal descent during breech birth assume the lithotomy position on a hospital delivery bed, and this is reflected in training simulations of breech delivery. As illustrated in Figure 6.1, women may be encouraged to adopt a semi-recumbent, adapted lithotomy position in the home environment. The mother will need to be on the end of the bed or settee so that her

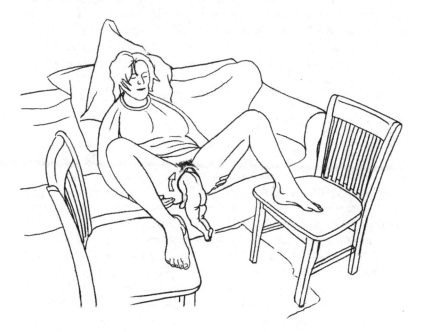

Figure 6.1 The semi-recumbent, adapted lithotomy position at home, showing the direction of the rotation used to free the arm during the Løvsets manoeuvre

bottom is at the edge and two chairs or people are needed to support the mother's legs.

'All fours' position – promoting physiological breech vaginal birth

Mothers with breech presentation may be encouraged to adopt an 'English pray' position. This appears to help the baby's trunk descend through the pelvis at a 45° angle and to move more naturally around the curve of the maternal pelvis. The mother kneels on the floor and leans up on to the bed or settee for support (Figure 6.2).

As described later, the 'all fours' position may then be adopted for the birth of the head using the Mauriceau–Smellie–Veit Manoeuvre (Figure 6.6). These manoeuvres are being explored by skilled midwives undertaking physiological breech births. Several midwives within the independent midwife circuit are attempting to explain and describe the mechanisms of this approach, and their findings from hands-on experience will hopefully be shared in the near future (Evans and Cronk 2003/04). It must be emphasised that skilled practitioners are the key to physiological vaginal breech births and these are unfortunately on the decrease. Jane Evans and Mary Cronk are presently organising nationwide 'sharing the skills' workshops to help rectify this situation.

The standing or squatting positions

The mother may wish to stand or squat. Remember that whilst gravity helps to expel the baby, it is the expulsive contractions and optimal position and angle of the maternal pelvis that facilitates a physiological breech birth. Although midwives have done standing breeches, the perinatal outcomes associated with this approach, reported in small numbers, have not been favourable (Steer 2002, Lewis 2002).

As most practitioners do some form of skills drills about breech birth in the lithotomy position (ALSO UK and others), it is necessary to describe this in the home context. Owing to a scarcity of skill in the community, the management of breech birth with the mother in an adapted lithotomy as well as in the 'all fours' position is described. It is advisable to practice all the following manoeuvres in the different positions with a model doll and pelvis. It is also advisable to seek out expert practical sessions with skilled practitioners.

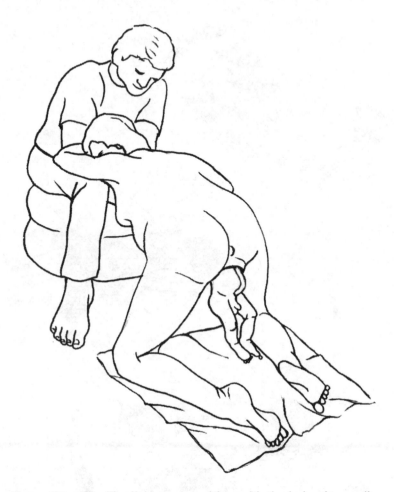

Figure 6.2   The 'English pray' position with the baby descending

The Løvsets manoeuvre to release extended arms

The Løvsets manoeuvre is used when either one or both arms are extended above the fetal head, obstructing labour if not released (Figure 6.3). This complication is recognised when, during the birth of the baby's trunk and chest, the arms fail to appear. The mother can be positioned either in an adapted lithotomy position or on all fours for this manoeuvre.

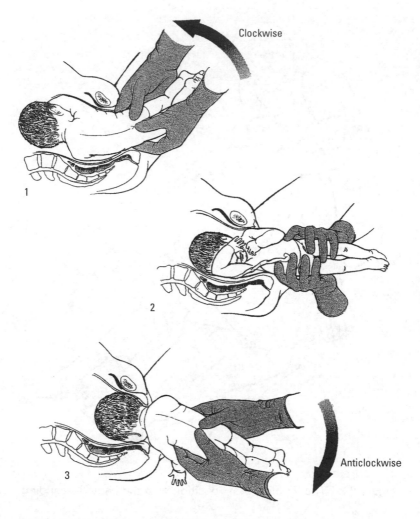

Figure 6.3 The Løvsets manoeuvre in the semi-recumbent/
lithotomy position

The Løvsets manoeuvre in the semi-recumbent position

1 The principles are simultaneous rotation and downward traction
   which enable delivery of the lower-lying arm first.
2 Hold the baby by the iliac crests, thumbs over sacrum, and, whilst
   applying gentle downward traction, rotate the baby 180 degrees

so that the baby's posterior arm, lying in the sacral curve, comes to lie anteriorly under the pubic arch. The anterior arm is delivered and the baby can then be rotated back the other way to deliver the second arm, if necessary (always keep the fetal back uppermost).

3　If the arm is not born spontaneously, then splint the humerus with two fingers, flex the elbow and sweep the arm downwards across the chest.

As can be seen in Figure 6.1, in an adapted lithotomy position the first arm has been delivered by the Løvsets manoeuvre, and the arrow indicates the direction the baby was rotated.

Løvsets manoeuvre in the 'all fours' position

In an emergency breech birth situation in the mother's home, you may meet this maternal position. In this position, because of the forces of gravity, traction is rarely needed and it is possible to release the arms in the same way as described above, if required. Make sure the baby's back remains facing the mother's front and take care to grasp the baby by the pelvic girdle to avoid soft tissue injury if you need to release arms and/or prevent rotation to a sacral posterior position. If the baby's left arm is trapped, then rotate the baby to the left in order to release the arm, and vice versa for the right if required.

Manoeuvres to deliver the aftercoming head

The Burns Marshall manoeuvre

This manoeuvre, now rarely performed in UK practice, facilitates movement of the head through the outlet and is only possible with the mother in a semi-recumbent, adapted lithotomy position. The fetus is allowed to 'hang' until the nape of the neck and subocciptal region is born. Grasp the ankles and, while maintaining traction to prevent the neck from bending backwards and resulting in possible cervical spine fracture, pivot the sub-occipital region under the pubic arch through an 180° arc until the mouth and nose are free of the vulva (Figure 6.4). Do this slowly to prevent undue pressure to the head and sudden stretching of the perineum. It is crucial that the baby is allowed to descend sufficiently before undertaking this manoeuvre to ensure that it is the suboccipital

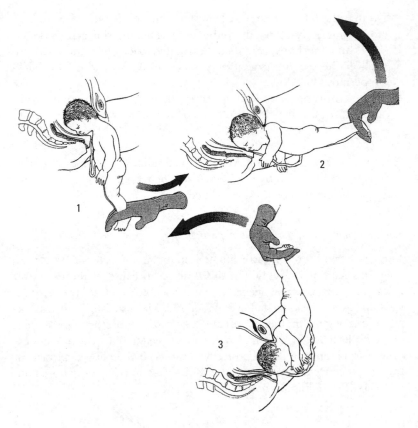

Figure 6.4   The Burns Marshall manoeuvre

region and not the neck that pivots under the pubic arch. If done too early, fracture of the cervical vertebra and crushing of the spinal cord may occur.

The Mauriceau–Smellie–Veit manoeuvre

The preferred manoeuvre is the Mauriceau–Smellie–Veit (Figure 6.5) which facilitates the birth of the head through the same arc but gives more control and places less strain on the fetal neck. This manoeuvre can be done in the semi-recumbent, adapted lithotomy position or with the mother in the 'all fours' position (described later). The

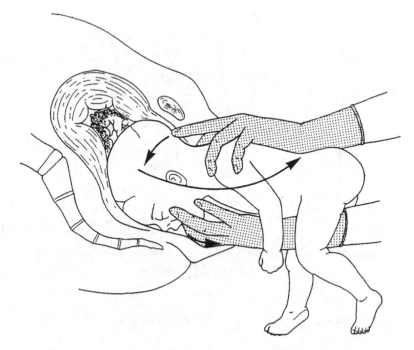

Figure 6.5 The Mauriceau–Smellie–Veit manoeuvre in the semi-recumbent/lithotomy position

manoeuvre facilitates maximum flexion of the fetal head and is often used when the fetal head is extended and descent is delayed. It also permits slow delivery of the head. With the mother in the semi-recumbent position:

1 Support the baby on one of your arms with your first and ring fingers placed on the baby's cheek bones, pulling the jaw down and increasing flexion (to avoid injury as referred to earlier, do not insert the middle finger in the baby's mouth).

2 Place the other hand across the baby's shoulders with your middle fingers on the occiput to increase flexion. The outer fingers can also gently apply traction to the baby's shoulders.

3 The head is delivered until the suboccipital region appears.

4 Pivot the baby's head gently and slowly around the symphysis pubis, delivering the chin and face first.

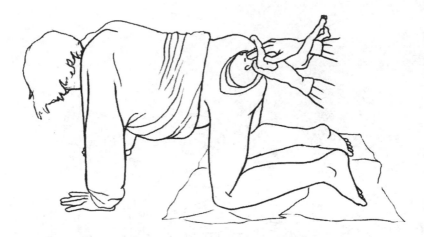

Figure 6.6   The adapted Mauriceau–Smellie–Veit manoeuvre
in the 'all fours' position

Breech birth in the 'all fours' position

The baby is born by contractions and maternal effort. The baby will then birth by expulsive contractions around the pelvic arc in the 'all fours' position, providing an excellent view of the birth process while it is happening and access to the baby's face as it is born over the perineum (Cronk 1998).

If the head fails to deliver spontaneously and promptly, you may need to flex the baby's head by tipping the occiput forwards with the middle finger of your right hand and by gentle pressure to the baby's cheek-bones with the fingers of your left hand. In effect, the Mauriceau–Smellie–Veit manoeuvre upside down (Figure 6.6). The vault of the baby's head should be born slowly and gently to facilitate gradual adaptation of the head to the changing pressures imposed by the birth process.

Vaginal breech birth: important practice points

- Because the fetal body is able to pass through the cervix prior to full dilatation, the mother may experience a premature urge to push. It is therefore vital always to check for full dilatation before encouraging the mother to push, to avoid the fetal head becoming entrapped in the partially dilated cervix. This could result in asphyxia and perinatal morbidity and mortality, as explained earlier.

- From the birth of the bitrochanteric diameters (the baby's hips) until full birth, no more than 15 minutes should elapse (Stevenson 1993). These are approximate timings that have not undergone any systematic scrutiny.

- As the body delivers, loosen the umbilical cord gently if needed (*rarely* required) to avoid spasm and constriction of the blood vessels. The cord can be used to feel for the fetal heart along with observing the chest movements (easier in the 'all fours' position). The fetal heart rate occasionally slows as a possible autonomic reflex in order to conserve oxygen in the fetal system as the uterus surface area reduces (Stevenson 1993).

- If the fetus enters the pelvis in a sacroposterior position, labour may become obstructed and delivery may be difficult. The head enters the pelvis in an occipitoposterior position where the occiput moves into the hollow of the sacrum, causing the head to deflex and increasing the diameters. This is very unusual and should be prevented. If the fetus is presenting or rotating to the sacral posterior, gently encourage it to maintain the anterior position or manually rotate back to the sacral anterior if necessary by holding the pelvic girdle, being careful not to damage fetal internal organs.

- No more than five minutes should pass from birth of the body to birth of the head because of cord compression and the high risk of hypoxia. Although no conclusive evidence exists, it is recommended that approximately three minutes be taken to deliver the vault of the fetal skull to avoid rapid decompression which may result in intracerebral haemorrhage.

- Although it is preferable to allow the baby to be born by gravity and with minimum handling (a physiological birth), it is essential to be aware of and skilled in manoeuvres to assist the breech-presenting baby if problems arise with the progress of labour and fetal descent and to control the birth of the fetal head.

- However, and most importantly, do not perform breech extraction (routine use of manoeuvres and interventions to expedite delivery). If you pull a breech baby down through the pelvis it is likely to cause delay and obstruction to the birth process. The fetal arms will be pulled upwards and the head extended backwards so that the occiput moves towards the fetal back leading to nuchal arm(s) and a hyper-extended head that can jeopardise the safety of the birth process and consequent health of the infant. Breech babies should birth by propulsion as a result of uterine contractions NOT traction. If the breech is not descending, it is necessary to transfer in to the hospital for Caesarean section. The rule is 'keep your hands off' a breech that is birthing spontaneously.

Other practice issues

The decision whether or not to advise transfer into hospital

Planned home birth

During a planned home birth, Caesarean section will be necessary if labour does not progress satisfactorily. Progress of labour is monitored by noting fetal descent on abdominal palpation, increasing regularity and duration of contractions, pain/pressure in the pelvic region, changes in the woman's behaviour and breathing, and changing emotional states (Burvill 2002). A vaginal examination, if indicated, provides additional information on position, station, dilatation of the cervix, and membranes, and adds to the assessment of labour progress. If no progress is occurring at home, inform the local consultant obstetrician, call an ambulance and calmly transfer in to hospital for Caesarean section. Unless there is fetal compromise there is no 'emergency or concern'.

Unplanned home breech birth

In the situation where hospital birth has been arranged and you are called to a woman in labour at home, it is important to undertake a careful assessment of the physical risk to mother and baby and the parent's wishes before deciding whether or not to transfer in to hospital. Once this assessment is made, based on the stage of labour, the position of the baby, and maternal medical and obstetric history, a plan of care with explicit rationale can be made. For example, you arrive at the home, the mother wants to push, and there is anal dilatation – it would be safer to proceed with the birth at home while calling for assistance rather than attempt a transfer in an ambulance. Assisting a woman to birth her breech baby in the back of an ambulance with little room and a cold ambient temperature is not the safest of options.

If you do need to transfer, then be prepared for the birth. Ensure that the receiving hospital knows why you are coming. Ensure that the paramedics are equipped for neonatal resuscitation, and continue to monitor the fetal heart and maternal condition whilst documenting findings during the journey. Take several towels in which to wrap the baby if it is born en route. Remember skin-to-skin contact for warmth. If the birth progresses more quickly than anticipated, consider asking the ambulance to shop, in order to undertake any necessary manoeuvres safely and effectively.

Monitoring the fetal heart and wellbeing

Inadequate monitoring in labour was emphasised in the CESDI 7th Annual Report (2000) on breech outcomes. Regular fetal heart monitoring should be employed and documented. Intrapartum fetal surveillance is shown to be critical in avoiding fetal death. Although the National Institute for Clinical Excellence (NICE 2001) guidelines recommend continuous electronic fetal heart monitoring for breech birth, in the home situation the midwife is advised to maintain close surveillance on the fetal heart patterns. This can be through Pinard or Sonicaid auscultation every 15 minutes during and following a contraction in the first stage, and following each contraction in the second stage of labour. The base-line rate, along with variability of at least ten beats per minute, and accelerations and decelerations should be noted. However, the timings of these auscultations are only a guide; no conclusive evidence exists to promote any strict guidance on intermittent auscultation but those stated here are now used as good practice.

If the membranes rupture and the buttocks are not well engaged into the pelvis, it would be advisable to check for cord prolapse. If there is cord presenting, then treat as for cord prolapse with a cephalic presenting baby. If a footling breech is discovered, ensure the cervix is fully dilated to allow descent and birth of the rest of the baby. It is common to get thick meconium at a breech birth owing to abdominal compression and this is not in itself a cause for concern. It is often described as being of 'toothpaste' consistency. In most cases the meconium is not in the amniotic fluid and is isolated to below the presenting buttocks. However, immediate suction of the oropharynx and inspection of the vocal cords will be required if the baby has thick meconium in the mouth and is not responsive at birth.

Care of the baby after birth

In order to avoid thermal shock, be prepared with warm towels and a warm ambient temperature without draughts for the birth itself. Consider having a heated warm pad that the baby can be laid on for examination and/or resuscitation. Have the heating put on and drape some towels over radiators. You may have to wrap the baby in a warm towel while awaiting completion of the birth process if the ambient temperature is cool. However, it is better to raise the ambient temperature and keep your hands off.

After the birth the woman's skin temperature will help, or that of her birth partner if this is not possible. Skin-to-skin contact will also facilitate breast-feeding which itself improves the baby's temperature. Remember that a baby who required resuscitation and/or who gets cold would be at greater risk of hypoglycaemia, and feeding should be a priority in the immediate postnatal period (Resuscitation Council (UK) 2001).

Preparation for neonatal resuscitation

Always be prepared for neonatal resuscitation. More breech babies are born requiring some resuscitation than cephalic-presenting births. If you are a midwife or general practitioner at home, consider calling the paramedics to wait outside, especially if the breech is undiagnosed and the woman's history is unknown.

Management of the third stage of labour

Management of the third stage is no different from that of a vertex delivery. The options for active management or physiological birth of the placenta remain determined by maternal choice, safety and appropriateness of the chosen method and situation. For example, a precipitate breech birth without a 'birthing kit' available that includes Oxytocic drugs would necessitate a physiological approach. This involves leaving the cord intact until complete birth of the placenta then clamping and cutting. If the baby requires resuscitation and there is no room available within the length of cord, then the cord needs to be clamped and cut. It is important then to unclamp the maternal end of the cord to facilitate physiological separation of the placenta. However, if undertaking an active management of the third stage, the maternal end should remain clamped.

Ensuring a conducive environment

These principles apply to both the emergency and the planned scenarios. Continuity of care throughout the childbearing process from a knowledgeable companion enhances the physiological process of giving birth (Hodnett 2000). The environment should be conducive to enhancing physiological processes: quiet and safe, with dimmed light and an avoidance of fear-inspired language. Remember that if the woman becomes frightened and unduly stressed, adrenaline levels increase and work against the effects of Oxytocin, leading to both more pain and dystocic labour (Odent 1999). The effects of this can then cascade into third stage resulting in bleeding, and even breast-feeding can be adversely affected. An understanding of the interplay of hormones is imperative for a birth attendant who wishes to promote the dynamic physiological processes safely. Owing to the increased statistical risk of fetal health problems, it would appear wise to avoid opiates for maternal analgesia and Oxytocin to force the baby through the pelvis.

Care of family members/friends at birth

The family may be very traumatised by the events unfolding. You yourself, as the health professional, may feel insecure and anxious, but you need to remain in control of the situation and provide direction and support to those involved. Anyone present at a birth may be called upon to help in an emergency: lay person, student or colleague. It is up to the lead professional to organise and initiate, giving directions to the team involved. You may have to arrange for the partner to leave the room if he panics, accompanied by someone if available. Siblings do not often become distressed unless they sense that the 'adults' are. Be aware of the effects on young minds in an emergency situation in their own home; they could become very frightened.

Documentation

Documentation is imperative. Document all discussions and referrals in full as they occur. Be specific about what is discussed in your notes. If events are moving quickly and you are alone, write in note form and transcribe later with the heading 'Retrospective notes written at (actual time of writing) from summary notes taken at the time'. Document the following clearly:

- Time of initial assessment: breech diagnosis, stage of labour with a clear plan of action and advice given.
- Time of assistance/referrals requested, who they are and the time they arrive.
- Plan for appropriate place of birth (woman's choices are also to be documented).
- Fetal heart rate with Sonicaid in the home between each contraction in second stage of labour.
- Position of mother, position of baby.
- Time presenting part seen at vulva; what it is.
- Time buttocks born and colour of skin.
- Time baby is born to umbilicus and colour of skin; any manoeuvres used.
- Time baby is born to neck, arms out and colour of skin; any manoeuvres used.
- Time baby is completely born; any manoeuvres used.
- Immediate condition of baby and resuscitation details (if needed).

Keeping in contact

The community staff needs excellent communication networks. Lists of phone numbers on the client's notes, along with detailed instructions on how to get to the home, need to be on the front of the notes. Staff must carry a mobile phone that can be charged constantly in the car between visits. A pager is also recommended as a necessary back-up communication between community staff. It is no good if the second midwife's phone is flat or out of range when called in an emergency. The midwife should ensure that the mobile phone stays with her wherever she is working in the client's home. It is no good if the phone is downstairs when you first see the buttocks being born. Leave the front door ajar so that you do not need to leave the mother.

Dignity and privacy

It is important that the woman is in control and maintains her dignity and privacy. It is good practice to have two practitioners at a breech vaginal birth. Other practitioners such as the paediatrician should be available in the hospital environment. With the rareness of breech vaginal births, people often want to come and 'watch'. Ensure that the room does not fill with spectators other than those whom the woman has given her consent to be there. This applies to both home and hospital.

Post-incident care

Most health professionals and parents expect a positive outcome. Sometimes, as with the unplanned breech birth, normal coping mechanisms are challenged. The unexpectedness of the situation, coupled with the lack of time to discuss options, may leave all involved potentially traumatised. There is some evidence to suggest that poor bonding, feeding problems, depression and post-traumatic stress disorder can ensue as a result of a breech birth experience (Albrechtsen et al. 1998). It is important that all involved have time to go through the events of the birth and to meet with the family to discuss the events of the birth. It is best to be honest and clear so that all involved are not left ambiguous about the events as they saw them.

Training issues

Breech vaginal birth has largely been neglected in midwifery training owing to increases in Caesarean sections for breech and a loss of skills amongst mentors now facilitating student midwives in the clinical areas. Paramedics and community midwives in particular, should practise their breech birth skills. Community midwives should have on-going skill drills with life-size dummies in the home environment once or twice a year. This is in addition to regular neonatal resuscitation skill updates on resuscitation dolls. Experienced breech vaginal birth practitioners need to run local and national workshops to avoid total loss of these skills in the midwifery profession. Most midwives have access to a doll and pelvis and can go through the breech mechanism and possible manoeuvres on a regular basis. These short sessions in small groups are highly effective in maintaining the mechanical skills involved. This is especially pertinent to the community-based staff, who could be assisting at a breech on their next on-call.

Supervisor of midwives' commentary

Midwives working in the community could be called to an unplanned 'normal' home birth at any time. It may cause a modicum of excitement, but it should be considered to be all in a day's work.

However, if the same midwife attended the same home to discover the pending birth was a breech presentation, she might experience considerably more than a modicum of excitement. Many midwives have very limited, if any, experience of a vaginal breech delivery due to increased hospitalisation and medicalisation over the years, and the current practice of delivering breech-presenting fetuses by elective Caesarean section.

As we already know, the unexpected will happen. It is therefore of paramount importance that midwives and obstetricians practise 'skills and drills' in the workplace and attend emergency scenario workshops in order to refresh on the theory as well as the practical procedures. This yearly update is the minimum amount of preparation required, and midwives would benefit from reading then rereading chapters such as this one and regularly practising delivery techniques alone or within clinical supervision sessions.

As well as the scenario of being faced with an unplanned breech delivery, you may find yourself preparing for a planned home breech delivery. Thorough preparation is essential, remembering the following key points:

1 Confirm the breech presentation. This may include an appointment with an obstetrician.
2 Seek support from your supervisor of midwives; you may wish for her (him) to visit the parents at home with you to discuss the birth.
3 If this delivery is against professional advice, then set a time to discuss the birth with the mother. Try to explore her reasons for wanting to deliver her baby at home; if she has particular fears or concerns, then these may be adequately addressed prior to the delivery.
4 Agree a birth plan which clearly states the circumstances in which the mother will accept transfer in to the hospital.
5 Ensure that you can demonstrate clear, concise documentation of the discussions held, including the explanation of potential risks for the fetus and mother.

6   Demonstrate up-to-date training in the management of a breech delivery.

Obstetric commentary

Breech presentation occurs when the fetus presents with buttocks or feet first, which can create a mechanical problem in delivery of the fetus. The buttocks and feet of the fetus do not provide an effective wedge to block and dilate the cervix. The umbilical cord, therefore, may prolapse, and/or the head may get trapped during delivery. Predisposing factors include prematurity, placenta praevia, fibroids, bicornuate uterus and fetal anomalies. There are three types of breech presentation:

1   Frank (65 per cent): the hips of the fetus are flexed, and knees are extended.
2   Complete (10 per cent): the hips and knees of the fetus are flexed.
3   Incomplete (25 per cent): the feet (footling) or knees of the fetus are the lowermost presenting part.

The perinatal mortality attributable to vaginal delivery of breech presentation varies between two to four times that of cephalic presentation when corrected for abnormalities. Breech presentation is, therefore, considered as high risk by most obstetricians. On the other hand, some midwives believe that breech presentation is a variation of normal labour, and not an abnormal situation. As quoted in the text, the Confidential Enquiry into Still-births and Deaths in Infancy *7th Annual Report* (CESDI) reported that the single and most avoidable factor in causing stillbirths and deaths among breech babies is suboptimal care given in labour and leading to hypoxia. This is contrary to the widely held belief that birth trauma, caused by the conduct of delivery, is responsible for the excess risk.

The Term Breech Trial (TBT) ended the debate about the best route of breech delivery in favour of planned Caesarean section (CS). As highlighted in this chapter, this conclusion has not been to everybody's satisfaction. However, despite the criticism about its methodology, the TBT remains the largest randomised controlled trial to study what would happen in real life to most breech babies. Whether the health profession or women agree with the trial or not, it has led to the increasing use of CS as an elective mode of breech delivery in the UK.

Even with a trend towards elective Caesarean delivery of most breech babies, obstetricians as well as midwives and paramedics can face a situation where they are required to manage breech birth. In the CESDI review, a fifth of all the babies were born at home, many of them already delivering by the time a health professional attended. The unexpected nature of these events emphasises the need for explicit plans for dealing with an undiagnosed breech at home. Not all midwives or paramedics will have the opportunity for hands-on experience; structured simulated training courses such as ALSO (Advanced Life Support in Obstetrics) or MOET (Managing Obstetrics Emergencies and Trauma) should, therefore, be made available for all staff who may encounter a vaginal breech delivery.

External cephalic version (ECV) can reduce the CS rate for breech by 50 per cent, as it reduces the incidence of breech presentation at term.

The chapter provided details of spontaneous breech birth (described as physiological birth) as well as different manoeuvres of breech delivery. The difference between breech extraction and assisted vaginal delivery was not made clear and could be identified as follows:

- Assisted vaginal delivery which is commonly practised in most hospitals and often includes epidural analgesia, artificial rupture of the membranes, lithotomy position, routine episiotomy, and different manoeuvres to deliver the legs and arms as well as the head.
- Breech extraction, which is only performed to deliver a breech second twin, involves in addition inserting a hand to grasp a foot and pull on it to deliver one leg followed by the other. Total breech extraction for the singleton breech is associated with a 25 per cent incidence of birth injuries and a mortality rate of approximately 10 per cent.

CS is recommended for the footling breech, hyperextended head (diagnosed by scan), and expected big baby (over 4000 g). CS should also be considered in labour if there is lack of progress, high breech in the second stage or an abnormal fetal heart rate.

Key points

- Vaginal breech delivery simulated training is recommended.
- Babies in the breech position are at higher risk than cephalic babies.
- Not all breeches can or should be born vaginally.
- Exclude factors that may not favour a spontaneous vaginal breech birth.
- 'Hands off the breech' is the golden rule for managing breech births. Damage is more often done by exerting too much force than by the baby being stuck.
- If there is delay during labour, or a complication arises, transfer the woman to hospital and consider CS.

- Maintain adequate support to the woman at all times and keep a good record of labour and delivery progress.

A problem-based scenario and interactive action planning exercise
An emergency undiagnosed breech birth in the community

The labour ward manager has called the local community midwife to attend a woman having her second baby. She is in advanced labour, and is booked for a hospital birth but feels unable to travel. The husband has panicked and called the ambulance and the GP. You are first to arrive at the woman's home. You have never met her. The door is open and you call out. A man shouts back, 'We are upstairs. I think it's coming!' You have no time to go and get any equipment, you run upstairs and you can hear the woman pushing. She is on all fours leaning on the bed and groans, 'Don't expect me to move now.' There is a big bag of membranes bulging out between the vulva, with what appears to be thick meconium.

Make your clinical assessment – take five minutes to answer the following questions:

- *What do you do first? Provide a rationale to your actions.*

- *Do you need to contact anyone and why?*

- *What are your thoughts now?*

- *What are the mother's options at this stage?*

The membranes rupture; thick meconium falls in lumps on to the floor. You see what you imagine is the anterior buttock.

- Practise a breech birth – use a doll and pelvis
- Describe in detail your actions up until the buttocks are fully born.
- When would you intervene to assist the infant's birth? Think about whether the baby has its back to the maternal abdomen or maternal spine.
- What manoeuvres, if any, do you use? Why do you use them? If the baby is sacral posterior what is the problem?

The baby is born up to the chest but the arms are not coming.

- Explain why you **would not** apply traction to the coming body. If you did what would happen?
- Describe how you will release the arms, using the doll and pelvis.

The baby continues to emerge until the nape of the neck is seen. The baby is hanging with gravity but minutes pass and the head is not coming.

- Describe how you will help the head to be born. Use the doll and pelvis. Differentiate between hands off and the need for hands on – write down your rationale.
- At what point would you initiate the manoeuvres? How long can the head not be delivered for?
- Think about the position – she is in on all fours. What manoeuvre would you use to help the head birth gently?

The baby is born 10 minutes after you arrive; he is 4.2 kg. The first Apgar is only 5; you need to resuscitate. At 5 minutes he improves with an Apgar of 7. Help arrives. At 10 minutes the Apgar is 10

- What are your priorities for the baby following the birth?
- Describe your documentation of the birth. Also think through the issues for the parents in this situation following the birth.

A possible action plan for this scenario

- The baby is going to be born soon; it is not possible to transfer safely.
- Call for help if this has not already arrived.
- Reassure the mother and other birth attendants; explain what is happening.
- Get someone to make the room warm, close windows and doors, and put the heating on if possible.
- Get warm towels and put them over the radiator for the baby.
- Send someone to get 'birth equipment' from the car (if you have some).

- Prepare the area for the baby and neonatal resuscitation, including suction.
- Ask someone to make notes of the times and the unfolding scenario for later documentation.
- Explain that thick meconium is common with breech babies and is not usually a problem (be prepared for suction if the baby has thick meconium in the mouth and is not responsive at birth).
- Allow the mother to adopt or remain in the position that feels most comfortable – in this case on her knees leaning on to the bed.
- Monitor the baby's heart after each contraction and record the time and the heart rate.
- Observe constant progress. The baby should increasingly descend and emerge with each contraction.
- Ensure that the baby remains in a sacro/occipito anterior position (gently rotate the baby to anterior if it begins to rotate to the posterior). Do not apply traction as nuchal arms and a hyperextended head can be caused.
- If the arms do not come and the birth is not progressing, release the arms using the Løvsets manoeuvre. Do not press on the baby's abdomen; hold the baby by the pelvic bones. Rotate the baby to one side so that the posterior arm sweeps over the front of the baby changing it to the anterior and can be released by folding the arm at the elbow. Repeat for the other arm if required. Ensure that the baby remains sacral anterior.
- If the head is not coming, consider using the Mauriceau–Smellie–Veit to flex the head and gently apply traction, delivering the head around the arc of the pelvis. Do this slowly.
- Initiate neonatal resuscitation by first drying the baby and maintaining warmth, stimulus, suction and facial oxygen. Use a bag and mask if still not responsive (see Chapter 7). Feed as soon as possible.
- Document and discuss events with all concerned.

References

Albrechtsen S, Rasmussen S and Dalaker K (1998) Reproductive Career After Breech Presentation: Subsequent Pregnancy Rates, Intrapregnancy Interval and Recurrence, *Obstetrics and Gynaecology* **92** (3), 345–50.

Allison J (1996) *Delivered at Home*. Chapman and Hall: London.

Banks M (2002) *Breech Birth Beyond the Term Breech Trial*. www.birthspirit.co.nz/termtrial.htm, accessed 17/7/02 see p. 208.

Barrett J (1991) Funic Reduction for the Management of Umbilical Cord Prolapse, *American Journal of Obstetrics and Gynaecology* **165**, 654.

Burvill S (2002) Midwifery Diagnosis of Labour-Onset, *British Journal of Midwifery* **10** (10), 600–5.

CESDI (Confidential Enquiry into Stillbirth and Death in Infancy) *7th Annual report* 2000 *Confidential Enquiry into Stillbirths and Deaths in Infancy* Maternal and Child Health Research Consortium London.

Coates T (1999) Malpositions of the Occiput and Malpresentations. In V R Bennett, and L K Brown (eds), *Myles Textbook for Midwives* (5th edn). Churchill Livingstone: Edinburgh.

Confino E, Gleiecher N, Elrad H, Isajovich B and David M P (1985) The Breech Dilemma. A Review, *Obstetrical and Gynecological Survey* **4** (6), 330–7.

Cronk M (1998) Midwives and Breech Births, *Practising Midwife* **1** (7), 44–5.

DoH (Department of Health) (1993) *Report of the Expert Maternity Group 'Changing Childbirth'*. HMSO: London.

DoH (Department of Health) (2000) *The NHS Plan*. The Stationery Office: London.

Evans J and Cronk M (2003/04) Personal Communication.

Hannah M and Hannah W (1996) Caesarean Section or Vaginal Birth for Breech Presentation at Term, *British Medical Journal* **312**, 1433–4.

Hannah M, Hannah W, Hewson S, Hodnett E, Saigal S and Willan A (2000) Planned Caesarean Section versus Planned Vaginal Birth for Breech presentation at Term: A Randomised Multicentre Trial, *Lancet* **356**, 1375–83.

Hawkey M (1997) Acupuncture: An Alternative Option in Pregnancy, *British Journal of Midwifery* **12** (12), 40–2.

Hodnett E (2000) *Caregivers Support During Childbirth*. In *The Cochrane Library*, **Issue 1**, 2002 Update Software: Oxford.

Hofmeyr G J (1996) Cephalic Version by Postural Management. In M W Enkin, M J N C Keirse, M J Renfrew and J P Neilson (eds), Oxford Update Issue 3, *Pregnancy and Childbirth Module of the Cochrane Database of Systematic Reviews*. BMJ Publishing Group: London.

Hofmeyr G J and Kulier R (2004) External Cephalic Version for Breech Presentation at Term (Cochrane Review). In *The Cochrane Library*, **Issue 2** (most recent amendment 1999). John Wiley & Sons Ltd: Chichester.

Keirse M J N C (2002) Evidence-Based Childbirth Only for Breech Babies? *Birth* **29** (1): 55–9.

Lewis P (2002) Personal Communication.

Lowdon G (1998) Breech Presentation: Caesarian Operation versus Normal Birth, *AIMS Journal* **10** (3), 1–4.

Midwifery Today (1996) *Tricks of the Trade* (1), 10.

NICE (National Institute for Clinical Excellence) (2001) *The Use of Electronic Fetal Monitoring* Clinical Guideline C Series. NICE: London.

Nikodem V (1995) Upright vs Recumbent Position During First Stage of Labour. In M Enkin, M Keirse, M Renfrew and J Neilson (eds), *Pregnancy and Childbirth Module of the Cochrane Database of Systematic Reviews*. MJB Publishing Group: London.

Nwosu E, Walkinshaw S and Chia P (1993) Undiagnosed Breech, *British Journal of Obstetrics and Gynaecology* **100** (6), 534.

O'Cathain A, Walters S, Nicholl J, Thomas K and Kirkham M (2002) Use of Evidence Based Leaflets to Promote Informed Choice in Maternity Care: RCT in Everyday Practice, *British Medical Journal* **324**, 643.

Odent M (1999) *The Scientification of Love.* Free Association Books: London.

Oxorn-Foote H (1986) *Human Labour and Birth* (5th edn) Appleton-Century Crofts: New York.

RCOG (Royal College of Obstetricians and Gynaecologists) (1999) *Royal College of Obstetricians and Gynaecologists Green Top Guidelines: The Management of Breech Presentation: Guideline No. 20.* RCOG: London.

Resuscitation Council (UK) (2001) *Resuscitation at Birth – Newborn Life Support. Provider Course Manual.* Resuscitation Council (UK): London.

Robinson J (2000) Midwives Need Training in the Lost Art of Breech Birth, *British Journal of Midwifery* **8** (7), 447–50.

Robson S, Ramsey B and Chandler K (1999) Registrar Experience in Vaginal Breech Delivery. How Much is Occurring?, *Australian and New Zealand Journal of Obstetrics and Gynaecology* **39**, 215–7.

Roosmalen J V and Rosendaal F (2002) There is Still Room for Disagreement About Vaginal Delivery of Breech Infants at Term, *British Journal of Obstetrics and Gynaecology* **109**, 967–9.

Stapleton H, Kirkham M and Thomas G (2002) Qualitative Study of Evidence Based Leaflets in Maternity Care, *British Medical Journal* **324**, 639.

Stear P (2002) Personal Communication.

Stevenson J (1993) More Thoughts on Breech, *Midwifery Today* **26**, 24–5.

Term Breech Trial Newsletter, June 2000 **4** (6) http://www.utoronto.ca/miru/breech/9806news.pdf, accessed 25/11/98.

Thornton J and Hayman R (2002) Staff Experience in Vaginal Breech Delivery, *British Journal of Midwifery* **10** (7), 408–10.

UKCC (United Kingdom Central Council for Nursing, Midwifery and Health Visiting) (1998) *Midwives Rules and Code of Practice.* UKCC: London.

7

Neonatal Resuscitation in Community Settings

Glenys Boxwell

Introduction

> As unforeseen complications can occur in any birth, every mother should be
> encouraged to have her baby in a maternity unit where emergency facilities
> are readily available. (Maternity services Advisory Committee 1984).

Pregnancy and delivery are, in most circumstances, normal social and
physiological processes, yet childbirth has become hospital-centred in
'developed' societies. Over the past 60 years the proportion of births in
the home has fallen from 80 per cent in 1930 to 1 per cent in 1990
(Zander and Chamberlain 1999). However, in the past few years the
proportions have begun to rise again, with Chamberlain, Wraight and
Crowley (1999) suggesting that home birth may increase to 4 or 5 per
cent during the next decade. Safety for both the mother and the baby
should be the foundation of good midwifery practice, with care and
attention being given to both the risks and the benefits of choosing the
home as an appropriate place for birth. Studies in both the UK and
Europe suggest that home births are as safe as hospital births for 'low-
risk' women (Chamberlain, Wraight and Crowley 1999, Weigers et al.
1996, Ackermann-Liebrich et al. 1996, Davies et al. 1996).

Resuscitation at birth is a relatively frequent occurrence. Saugstad
(1998a) suggests that 3 to 5 per cent (four to seven million) of the 140
million newborn infants born worldwide each year need some kind of
resuscitation at the time of birth. Statistically, the need for resuscitation
in the newborn infant in the home setting is less than that of hospital

confinements (Chamberlain, Wraight and Crowley 1999). However, midwives and parents should not be lulled into a false sense of security with this data, and the planning of a home birth should incorporate contingency plans for dealing with a compromised infant. All midwives are mandated to 'examine and care for the newborn infant; to take all initiatives which are necessary in case of need and to carry out where necessary immediate resuscitation' (UKCC 1998 p. 26).

The latter part of that statement is particularly pertinent when one considers that 30 per cent of infants who require active resuscitation are delivered after an apparently normal labour in which there has been no evidence of fetal compromise (Roberton 1992). This statistic is a compelling reason for midwives delivering in the home environment to acquire and maintain the requisite skills and knowledge to undertake competently resuscitation manoeuvres that may be required of them.

Midwives and those attending home births need to understand the physiological asphyxial processes in order to rationalise interventions that may need to be undertaken for safe and effective resuscitation of the newborn.

This chapter will outline the physiology of asphyxia in order to set the context of resuscitative techniques, and will provide a practical guide to resuscitation in the home setting.

Asphyxia

The healthy fetus is equipped with protective mechanisms that allow it to withstand the rigours of labour and delivery, with its concomitant relative oxygen depletion, in order to prevent hypoxic organ damage. The high affinity for oxygen of fetal haemoglobin supports the diffusion of oxygen to the tissues, allowing oxygen extraction at tissue level to increase by almost 100 per cent during hypoxaemic events. This is due to a right shift of the haemoglobin oxygen dissociation curve (decreased affinity), which enhances oxygen extraction, delaying the development of hypoxic damage (Bocking et al. 1992, Talner et al. 1992).

Additionally, differences in the fetal heart compared to that of an adult assists in reducing hypoxic tissue damage. The fetal heart rate is a major determinant of cardiac output, as it is four times greater than that of an adult per kilogram body weight, owing to the combined output of right and left ventricles, 50 per cent of this output directed to the placenta and increasing the placental oxygen uptake (Cohn et al. 1974).

The combination of these mechanisms allows for a wide safety margin of adequate oxygen delivery during labour. In short-duration hypoxaemic events, the mature fetus's heart rate will fall but, as it is associated with an increase in arterial blood pressure, myocardial contractility is increased and cardiac output is maintained. This is the result of vascular resistance changes in the fetal gut, skin and muscle, which divert the blood supply to the heart, brain and adrenals (Cohn et al. 1974). This autoregulatory process is modulated at cellular level via the metabolic feedback regulation of the calibre of the arterioles and capillary sphincters (Grainger et al. 1975, cited in Talner et al. 1992). The heart and brain are efficient at autoregulation and can maintain their blood flow over a wide range of perfusion pressures and oxygen contents. Hypoxaemic events of this type are intermittent during labour, and the fetus's ability quickly to redistribute oxygenated blood is very important.

When there is no stress, the fetal and newborn heart is working at close to capacity merely to satisfy normal demands of tissues and growth (Talner et al. 1992). Any increased output requirement to satisfy suboptimal tissue oxygen demand cannot, therefore, be sustained for long and myocardial contractility will fail. So, whilst the fetus can make circulatory adjustments to compensate for the process of labour, under severe conditions these adaptive mechanisms will be overwhelmed, the shunting of the blood towards vital organs and cerebral oxygen delivery will reduce as the blood pressure and cardiac output fall, resulting in asphyxial injury.

There are five basic causes of asphyxia during labour and delivery:

1   Interruption of umbilical blood flow (for example, cord compression).
2   Failure of gas exchange across the placenta (for example, placental abruption).
3   Inadequate perfusion of the maternal side of the placenta (for example, severe maternal hypotension).
4   An otherwise compromised fetus who cannot tolerate the transient, intermittent hypoxia of normal labour (for example, the anaemic or growth-retarded fetus).
5   Failure to inflate the lungs and complete the change in ventilation and lung perfusion that must occur at birth (for example, obstructed airway or poor or absent respiratory effort) (Phibbs 1994).

Levene (1995 p. 405) encapsulates these causes in his definition of asphyxia as 'the impairment of placental or pulmonary gas exchange resulting in hypoxaemia, hypercarbia and acidosis'.

The ability of an organ to maintain aerobic metabolism is dependent upon:

- the amount of oxygen delivered to the tissue;
- the amount of oxygen extracted by the tissue; and
- the amount of metabolic energy in the form of adenosine triphosphate (ATP) required.

When oxygen delivery and blood flow diminish considerably, anaerobic metabolism (glycolysis) will result, becoming the supplementary mechanism to maintain cellular energy stores. This glycolysis is a short-term emergency measure, which produces just one-fifteenth of the ATP that would be produced aerobically and, as a consequence, utilises stored glucose (glycogen) very rapidly. The resultant production of pyruvate and lactate leads to a gradual accumulation of lactate in the blood and tissues, leading to a metabolic acidaemia. ATP is required to maintain the ion gradient of sodium and calcium across the cellular membrane. Failure of this mechanism leads to an influx of sodium and calcium in to the cells, which allows for an influx of water leading to intracellular swelling. This acute swelling creates cytotoxic cerebral oedema, which may contribute to brain injury.

As birth asphyxia is arguably the most common cause of perinatally acquired severe brain injury in the full-term infant (Levene 1995 p. 405), midwives practising in any setting have a responsibility to be able to ameliorate its potentially devastating effects by prompt and skilled resuscitation.

Preparation

The need for resuscitation is unpredictable, but a contingency plan should be in place in case it is necessary to implement it in an emergency.

Preparation begins with the booking interview, which Methven (1993) considers to be the most important aspect of midwifery care. During this interview, the place of birth should be discussed and any risk issues identified that may advise against a home delivery. The risks as well as the benefits of home deliveries should be highlighted, with specific reference to what may be required if the infant is compromised at birth. The woman needs to be made aware of the limited facilities and back-up the midwife has at home in the case of advanced resuscitation being required, and it would be negligent of the midwife not to make this information available.

It is reasonable to assume that, in the developed world, electricity and hot and cold water will be available but assumptions should not be made as to where in the home the woman is planning to deliver. The room needs to be assessed to ensure that it is adequately lit so that the infant can be properly assessed and it should have heating sufficient to keep the infant in optimal condition. Ideally (from the infant's perspective), the room should be warm, approximately 25°C if possible, with doors and windows closed to prevent draughts and convective heat loss. Thermal stability must be maintained if the infant is to be kept in good condition. The intrauterine environment is approximately 1.5°C greater than the maternal temperature. A newborn infant's temperature is approximately 37.8°C (range 37–39°C) (Mann 1968, cited in Rutter 1992). Potential heat losses by convection, radiation and evaporation will, therefore, be high, with the core temperature of a wet infant potentially dropping by 5°C in as many minutes (Milner 1995).

Cold stress is associated with hypoxia and acidosis which are factors that inhibit surfactant production in the newborn. If left unheeded, this situation will lead to respiratory distress, grunting and the potential for transfer to hospital.

As most midwives now carry mobile phones, the issue of summoning help, if required, should not pose a problem. However, some rural communities may have 'signal' problems and an available landline may be deemed necessary.

When the midwife arrives for the delivery, the equipment required for successful resuscitation should be laid out in an appropriate area beforehand (see Figure 7.1). All equipment should be regularly checked for signs of deterioration, and a safety check undertaken immediately prior to use. Whilst it may appear obvious that equipment is checked and suitable for the task, failure of this simple procedure is implicated in a number of neonatal deaths reported in the UK annually (CESDI 1995). The towels should be set to warm either on a radiator or by using a heat source or hot water bottle.

Immediate interventions

As soon as the infant delivers, the time should be noted and an assessment of the situation undertaken. The four parameters that need to be immediately assessed are colour, respiratory activity, heart rate and tone, as these will indicate what further course of action is needed.

Changing mat
Towels (at least three)
Stethoscope
Cord clamp
Self-inflating bag with pressure-limiting device (500 ml
   volume)
Facemasks size 0 and 1
Oxygen cylinder (full) (if Trust policy dictates the use of
   oxygen in home setting)
Suction device (battery and/or mains)
Suction catheters size 10 fg
Yankaeur sucker
Guedel airways size 0,00
Light source
Visible clock
Heat source, e.g. small mains mattress or hot water bottle
Emergency instruction cards (clearly printed), for example

Dial 999. Ask for emergency paramedic ambulance to be sent
   immediately to (address). Midwife/GP resuscitating infant.

Figure 7.1 Equipment required for successful
              neonatal resuscitation

Most healthy mature infants have spontaneous onset of respiration by ten seconds (Milner 1995) and no further assistance is required other than keeping the baby warm by careful drying, followed by skin-to-skin contact with the mother, with any exposed surfaces covered by dry, warm towels. It is vital that practitioners be mindful of the importance of temperature control and do not let other interventions take precedence, leaving the infant only partially dried, with wet hair, and in contact with damp towels.

An infant born in less than optimal condition requires further assessment. Place this infant onto a warmed, padded surface (changing mat covered in two warm towels), dry off immediately, removing the wet towel closest to the infant, and cover extremities, especially the head as it accounts for 25 per cent of the infant's surface area and is consequently a site for massive heat loss (Daze and Scanlon 1981). This intervention has the dual effect of reducing heat loss and providing tactile stimulation, which may be sufficient to induce gasping and onset of respiration.

Airway

Airway management is one of the most important steps in resuscitation and probably the least well managed (Resuscitation Council (UK) 2001a). An infant who has undergone any degree of compromise during the delivery process may be floppy at birth. This will affect not only the infant's general muscle tone, but also the tone of the airway. The lack of pharyngeal tone and the tongue becoming backwardly displaced will result in an obstructed airway. This situation is further compounded by the infant's relatively prominent occiput which, when the infant is placed supine on to a flat surface, results in flexion of the neck, bringing the head forward and creating a further structural obstruction. These obstructions are easily remedied by the manoeuvres recommended by the Resuscitation Council (UK) (2001b) of chin lift and jaw thrust (Figures 7.2 and 7.3).

During chin lift the midwife should place the middle finger on the bony tip of the infant's chin and bring the infant's head into the neutral position (whereby the nose is pointing directly upwards but not overextended). The use of a 2–3-cm thickness pad under the shoulders may be helpful in achieving and maintaining the head in a good position (Ziderman et al. 1998). If this manoeuvre in isolation is not sufficient to open the airway, then jaw thrust may be applied. This technique involves the use of one or two fingers being applied to the angle of the lower jaw, supporting the airway by lifting the jaw outwards and forwards. During both of these manoeuvres, care should be taken to ensure that the fingers are always on the bones of the infant's lower jaw and chin and not on the soft tissues of the underside of the jaw.

Once the structural obstruction is corrected, the infant may breathe spontaneously, but may require free-flow oxygen to correct any persisting cyanosis. This technique will also provide a cold stimulus to breathing (Ziderman et al. 1998) but what should be considered is that it can lead to significant cooling, which is counterproductive.

Persisting central cyanosis, apnoea or gasping, pallor or a heart rate less than 100 beats per minute (bpm) indicates the necessity for further intervention. The airway position should be reassessed and, once deemed established, then the process of initiating effective breathing for the infant should commence.

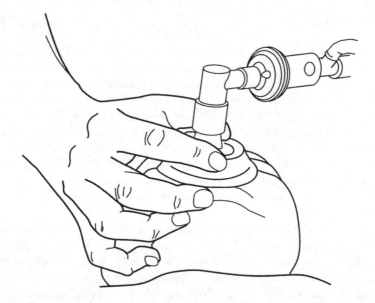

Figure 7.2 Jaw thrust and correct application of the face mask

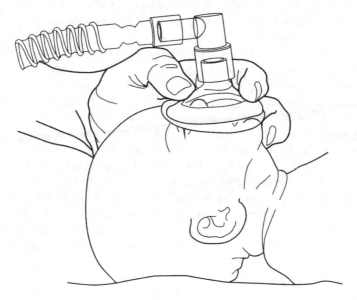

Figure 7.3 The correct mask position

Breathing

To establish regular respiration at birth, two processes need to occur: the removal of existing lung fluid and the visible movement of the infant's chest. This is achieved by application of an appropriate-sized face-mask. To size a face-mask the internal aperture should be sufficient to cover both the mouth and nose, with the external dimensions not covering the eyes or overhanging the chin. A circular mask with a soft, deformable cuff best provides this (Ziderman 1998, Resuscitation Council (UK) (2001b). The mask is effectively held in place by gripping its stem and applying gentle pressure; this technique avoids leaks around the periphery of the mask which can result in inadequate seal and poor chest movement (Figures 7.2 and 7.3).

Using a self-inflating bag with a volume of 500 ml and valve pop-off system of 30–40 cmH_2O, five slow inflation breaths should be given, attempting to sustain the inflation for two to three seconds. The sustained inflation will allow for achievement of the lungs, functional residual capacity (Vyas et al. 1981) and assist in forcing residual lung fluid into the pulmonary lymphatics. The chest should be visibly moving by the fifth inflation breath. The best way to monitor successful ventilation is to observe the chest movement and check the heart rate. The pulse will pick up quickly during a successful resuscitation procedure with at least three out of four asphyxiated infants having spontaneous breathing after these initial steps (Saugstad 1998a). If the chest is not moving, reassess the situation by checking the previously described manocuvres and repeat the process of five slow inflation breaths. Once the chest is moving, a breathing rate of 40 breaths per minute should be continued until the infant is breathing regularly for itself.

Currently the use of 100 per cent oxygen in newborn resuscitation is advocated (BMJ Working Party 1997, Chameides and Hazinski 1997, Ziderman et al. 1998, Resuscitation Council (UK) 2001b), although this may be considered controversial as there are potentially damaging effects. The term 'oxygen-free radical disease' has been introduced into newborn care in recent years, with the main emphasis of research being its association with complications of prematurity (Saugstad 1998b). These complications are thought to occur as a result of the premature infant's lack of antioxidant enzyme systems that counteract free radicals associated with the use of high oxygen concentrations (Sosensko 1995). The use of high concentration oxygen during the resuscitation of both premature and term infants could be debated. Lundstrom et al. (1995)

measured cerebral blood flow on premature infants who were resuscitated with either room air or 80 per cent oxygen. In the high oxygen group, cerebral vasoconstriction persisted, which, they concluded, might make the brain more susceptible to hypoxic episodes or ischaemia, thus potentially increasing the risk of cerebral damage in the newborn period.

Does a high inspired oxygen concentration during resuscitation detrimentally affect the term infant? In the term asphyxiated population, animal studies suggest high oxygen concentrations may also be damaging owing to hypoxia reperfusion injury. The animal studies of Rootwelt et al. (1992) and Raivio (1996) suggest that restoration of blood supply containing a high concentration of oxygen is more detrimental than restoration of the circulation alone as it appears to create radical oxygen metabolites which create further pathological changes. In the light of these findings, it is qustionable whether the recommendation that all infants be subjected to high oxygen concentrations at birth can be justified. More studies are required in this area to define best practice.

It should be also noted that, despite the above national recommendations that 100 per cent oxygen be used in neonatal resuscitation, not all community midwives carry oxygen to home births. Ramji et al. (1993) tested the hypothesis that room air was superior to 100 per cent oxygen by randomising 84 asphyxiated human newborns to receive either room air or 100 per cent oxygen. Of the 72 infants available for follow-up, none had adverse neurological sequela, suggesting that room air is as effective as oxygen in this setting. Saugstad et al. (1998) undertook a further study of this hypothesis concluding that asphyxiated newborn infants can be resuscitated with room air as effectively as with pure oxygen. Their findings also suggested that administration of 100 per cent oxygen appeared to depress ventilation, as the time to the first breath or cry was longer in this group.

Whilst the prevention of hypoxia must remain a high priority during neonatal resuscitation, the indiscriminate use of oxygen needs careful consideration in order to prevent potential long-term adverse sequelae.

Other airway manoeuvres

As suggested, the above techniques will be effective in gaining chest movement and establishing breathing *in most cases*. However, in the event that, despite a good technique, the chest does not move, adjunctive manoeuvres can be applied. The midwife needs to assess whether the airway is obstructed by particulate matter, that of meconium (there is usually external evidence of this!), blood clot or vernix. Clearance of the obstruction using controlled suction is advocated in this circumstance. As aggressive suction can induce severe bradycardia via vagal reflexes and laryngeal spasm, it needs to be undertaken as a controlled technique. Using a wide-bore catheter (10 fg) or Yankaeur sucker, careful and gentle suction should be applied to the oropharynx with the suction pressure limited to 100 mmHg (13.3 kPa) and the catheter advancing no further than 5 cm from the lips. The technique should take no longer than five seconds (Ziderman et al. 1998, Saugstad 1998a, BMJ Working Party 1997). Ideally, this technique is best undertaken by visualising the upper airway with the use of a laryngoscope; midwives who are trained and deemed competent in more advanced resuscitation techniques may choose to carry a laryngoscope with them to home births for this purpose. Once the particulate matter is removed, the inflation breaths should be repeated.

If the chest still does not move, the insertion of a Guedel airway may prove beneficial to further support the airway. The Guedel should be assessed to ensure it is the appropriate size for the infant. This is undertaken by holding it along the lower jaw with the flange directly below the infant's nose tip. The other end should be adjacent to the angle of the jaw. To insert the airway into an infant, insert it in the attitude in which it will lie, unlike the adult method where it is inserted into the mouth upside down and rotated (Resuscitation Council (UK) 2001a). This technique avoids potential trauma to the soft tissues of the mouth and upper oropharynx. The use of a Guedel airway is of great benefit in situations where more prolonged positive pressure ventilation may be required, and can provide for a more stable, secure airway during transfer of an infant in the absence of a person skilled in endotracheal intubation.

Circulation

Once the airway is patent and chest movement can be seen, the heart rate should be checked after approximately twenty to thirty seconds of good ventilation. This is most easily assessed in the newborn situation by palpation of the base of the umbilical cord. If a pulse cannot be palpated, auscultation of the chest must be undertaken. If the heart rate is less than 60 bpm, chest compressions should be commenced. There is no point in moving to chest compressions unless the chest is

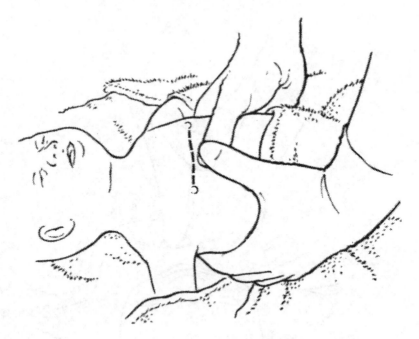

Figure 7.4   The two-thumb technique for chest compression

moving; if the infant is not being oxygenated, commencement of chest compressions is futile. This is optimally a two-person technique but can be adequately performed single-handed. There are two techniques described for cardiac compression in the newborn. The preferred technique is for the operator's hands to encircle the thorax, with the thumbs pointing towards the head rather than across the chest and placed side by side over the lower third of the sternum (Menegazzi et al. 1993, David 1988) (Figure 7.4). The sternum is then compressed to approximately one-third of the thorax depth (Chamedeis and Hazinski, 1997).

The compressions should be smooth and not jerky, with each one comprising 50 per cent compression and 50 per cent relaxation phases, to allow for adequate filling of the coronary arteries. To be most effective, the compressions should be interposed with a ventilation breath every third compression, as simultaneous chest compression may hinder ventilation. This 3:1 ratio will give 120 cycles per minute, for example

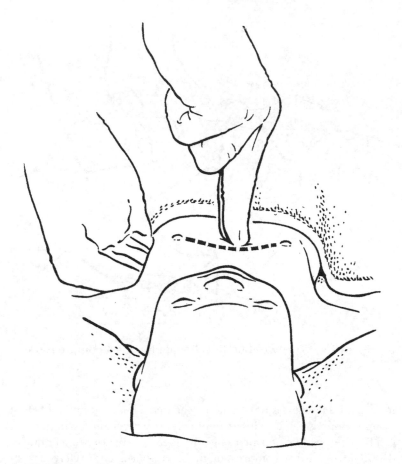

Figure 7.5   The two-finger technique for chest compression

90 cardiac compressions to 30 breaths. It is important that this rate is not exceeded, as too rapid cardiac compression will not allow for the relaxation phase of the procedure, which will hinder its effectiveness.

The alternative technique is to place the index and middle fingers on the lower third of the sternum and press at the same depth and rate as previously described (Figure 7.5). Whilst it is recognised that this technique is less effective in creating coronary artery perfusion pressures and mean arterial blood pressure than that previously described (Menegazzi et al. 1993), it may be more appropriate in the extremely low birth-weight population owing to the size of the thorax, or in a single-handed resuscitation situation.

Compressions should be stopped briefly every 30 seconds to check actual heart rate. Once the infant's spontaneous rate is above 60 and rising, compressions may stop. Ventilation breaths at 40 per minute should continue until the infant is breathing regularly.

Special cases

In the situation where the delivery becomes unexpectedly complicated, the woman should be immediately transferred to the nearest obstetric consultant unit by calling for an emergency ambulance. The midwife should telephone ahead to alert the clinical team of the expected time of arrival and the problems encountered. The midwife should accompany the woman in the ambulance during the transfer. However, if imminent transfer to hospital is not an option either because it would endanger the woman's safety or because the woman refuses to move, the midwife should:

- contact another midwife to attend (there is no legal requirement to provide two midwives to attend home births (RCM 2002) but in potentially complex situations it would be considered appropriate from a risk management perspective);
- contact the supervisor of midwives;
- contact the delivery unit to alert the medical team and senior midwife.

Meconium-stained liquor

Meconium-stained liquor occurs in 10 to 20 per cent of pregnancies at term (Halliday 1992). Whilst this incidence is high, the incidence of actual aspiration is said to be 5 per cent of infants in the USA (Wiswell and Bent 1993) and as few as 0.2 per cent of infants in the UK (Greenhough 1995).

Thick meconium is a marker of fetal hypoxia, the hypothesis being that in utero hypoxia increases intestinal peristalsis and relaxation of the anal sphincter tone. Aspiration is most likely to occur in utero owing to anoxic fetal gasping, and it is therefore a point of controversy as to how much benefit is gained from aggressive suctioning of the upper airway.

Following the delivery, the midwife needs to undertake an astute clinical assessment before deciding on the course of action to be taken; this initial assessment is of paramount importance.

The infant who then comes out vigorous and crying has an open, clear airway, and suction, with its potential concomitant complications, as described earlier, is unnecessary in this situation.

The infant who is delivered through meconium-stained liquor and who is floppy, with little or no respiratory effort and a low heart rate, is obviously compromised and requires immediate airway management as previously described. It is probably judicious in this situation to undertake suction of the upper airway as the first manoeuvre to remove any potential obstruction prior to giving inflation breaths.

When meconium is present at a delivery, there may be a tendency not to dry the infant thoroughly, based on the belief that drying the infant will stimulate breathing and cause the infant to aspirate meconium into the lungs. However, when thick meconium is in the infant's airway it is unlikely that it will be 'sucked down' into the lungs during drying, so, as with all infants, it should be gently and thoroughly dried as a first-line manoeuvre to lessen the likelihood of cold stress injury.

Other manoeuvres, such as cricoid pressure, epiglottal blockage and thoracic compression to prevent aspiration, are not recommended in the management of this situation. Not only are they not scientifically tested, they are also potentially dangerous as they can cause vagal stimulation, trauma and deep aspiration owing to chest recoil when the encircling hands are released.

Preterm infants

Infants born unexpectedly at home prior to term should be treated in exactly the same way as term infants with regard to resuscitation. As they are much more prone to thermal stress, careful attention needs to be given to drying the infant and covering its extremities. In the case of very preterm infants, i.e. less than 30 weeks, evidence exists that delivering them into a polythene bag is beneficial in the maintenance of body temperature in the hospital setting (Vohra et al. 1999, Björklund and Hellström-Westas 2000). This technique could easily be applied in the home situation. As soon as the infant is delivered, its entire body is put into the polythene bag (without drying), covering the back of the head but leaving the face exposed. The infant should then be put into prewarmed towels (referred to earlier) to reduce conductive heat losses, and further resuscitative manoeuvres can be performed with the infant inside the bag. Observation of chest movement can be visualised through the polythene bag. As in the hospital setting, it is recommended that the infant stay in the polythene bag for up to four hours, which is sufficient time for its emergency transfer from home to hospital to be arranged.

Preterm infants will require immediate transfer to hospital for on-going management. Telephoning for an emergency paramedic ambulance is the most expedient way of doing this as the organisation and liberation of a hospital-based neonatal 'flying squad' will take too long, requiring the infant to stay in a suboptimal environment for longer than is necessary. The nearest neonatal intensive care unit should be informed of the transfer so that they can be prepared for the infant's imminent arrival. In the presence of two midwives, one should accompany the infant to the hospital. If only one midwife is present, the continuing care of the infant should be transferred to the paramedic team.

Infants at the edge of viability

Since 1992 the age of viability of infants in the UK has been 24 weeks. However, Rennie (1996) uses the term 'marginal viability' when referring to infants of 23^{+0} to 26^{+6} weeks of pregnancy. She suggests that, as the prognosis for this group of infants is 50 per cent mortality, with 50 per cent of survivors being handicapped, there should be prenatal counselling of parents in order to discuss and formulate a plan for the resuscitation (or not) of the infant. In the absence of such a plan, as would be the case for a midwife called to this situation in the home, Rennie advocates that the best course of action is to attempt resuscitation in all live-born babies of 23 weeks and above.

Stillbirth

An infant delivered after the 24th week of pregnancy who has not at any time breathed or shown any signs of life is stillborn (UKCC 1998). The midwife who is present at the delivery of an unexpected stillbirth needs to assess the situation thoroughly as even infants apparently born dead can be successfully resuscitated and have a normal outcome. Casalaz et al. (1998) reported 42 cases of resuscitation in apparent stillbirth. When outcomes were analysed, 23 per cent of the surviving infants had severe disability, 36 per cent survived intact and a further 15 per cent were reported to have an 'equivocal outcome', with mild motor development problems but no developmental delay.

Consequently, resuscitation should be attempted unless signs of maceration are evident; this manifests as skin slipping which becomes apparent six to twelve hours after death (Berry 1992). If resuscitation is not successful, the stillbirth must be recorded by completion of a certificate of stillbirth. It is usual for a medical practitioner to issue the certification but a midwife who has personally witnessed the birth may do so. The midwife also needs to notify the supervisor of midwives. Discussions need to take place with the parents surrounding the issue of post-mortem examination of the stillbirth. If post-mortem examination is declined, tests such as glucose tolerance, Kleihaur and glycosylated haemoglobin (HbA$_1$C) should be suggested in order to try to elicit a cause and offer meaningful advice about subsequent pregnancies (CESDI 2001). If a post-mortem is to be undertaken, the midwife needs to ensure that any resuscitative attempts are clearly and precisely documented, as presence of air in the lungs may suggest that the infant breathed spontaneously and would be subsequently regarded as a live birth.

Unless clinically indicated, there is no real need for the woman to be transferred to hospital. The parents will require sensitive management at this time and need to be given practical advice surrounding the processes of registering the death and arranging a funeral. Giving contact details of both local and national support groups that are available may be useful to them. This information will be readily available in the local maternity unit or neonatal intensive care unit.

How long should resuscitation continue?

In the situation where prolonged resuscitation is thought to be necessary, for example in the case of a preterm infant, or where, despite best efforts and a good technique, the infant does not appear to be responding, any person who is available should be instructed to dial 999 and request a paramedic ambulance to attend immediately, giving the address and saying that the baby is being resuscitated by the midwife/GP. Recommendations suggest that resuscitation efforts should be discontinued if an infant has no cardiac output after ten to fifteen minutes, or if no respiratory effort is made by thirty minutes, when other factors for respiratory depression have been eliminated, for example opiate depression or neuromuscular disorders (Ziderman et al. 1998, Levene 1995). Hospital Trusts will have their own policies to determine when resuscitative efforts should be abandoned, with the most senior paediatrician or neonatologist available being called to make the final decision.

The midwife in the community setting does not have the luxury of this support network and is mandated to continue resuscitative techniques until either a medical practitioner arrives who is prepared to make the decision to stop, or until transfer to hospital for continued resuscitation or further intensive care manoeuvres can be arranged.

Prognosis following resuscitation

The prognosis of the term infant following an asphyxial insult is difficult to determine in the immediate post-delivery situation and can only really be predicted when the infant has been carefully assessed on the neonatal unit, when the degree of hypoxic ischaemic encephalopathy has been determined.

Prediction of outcome in asphyxiated infants is of obvious importance to parents, and the information needs to be given as clearly and honestly as possible. The prognosis can be more clearly and accurately given to parents if the appearance of the infant at birth and resuscitation manoeuvres are clearly documented. Following a resuscitation event, however minor or extensive, the interventions undertaken should be carefully and accurately documented. Record-keeping is an integral part of midwifery practice; it is not separate from the care-giving process and it is not an optional extra to be fitted in when circumstances allow (NMC 2002, UKCC 1998). The use of the numerical Apgar score alone is of little value, as infants with the same scores can have vastly differing aetiologies and therefore vastly different outcomes. Full written descriptors should accompany the scoring system if it is to be of any clinical value. Good documentation will allow for better continuity of care for the infant and parents, and foster improved communication and dissemination of information between members of the health care team.

Within documentation, the use of the term 'asphyxiated at birth' should be avoided, as any infant who fails to breathe spontaneously immediately at birth may not have undergone a hypoxic–ischaemic insult and the cause may not be immediately determined. The use of the term asphyxia may lead to misdiagnosis and cause controversies in the long term both medically and legally (Donn 1998).

Conclusion

The need for resuscitation at birth is unpredictable and, whilst women delivering in the home environment are usually considered 'low risk', the potential for the infant requiring some degree of intervention is always present. If the infants are to be given the best possible care in whichever setting they choose to deliver, midwives need to keep their skills up to date by attending practice-based refresher study days on techniques surrounding resuscitation, as deskilling occurs over time (Broomfield 1996).

A problem-based scenario and interactive action planning exercise Neonatal resuscitation following a home birth

Judy is a 23-year-old gravida 2 para 1, who has decided on a home delivery for her second child. Her first child Alfie was delivered in hospital two years ago and she 'didn't enjoy the experience'. She is fit and healthy and has had an unproblematic pregnancy.

In planning for this delivery what points and preparations need to be considered?

You have probably identified the following:

- Jane falls into a 'low risk' category.
- Home circumstances, e.g. the room she plans to delivery in has appropriate heating and lighting and a telephone, and there are good sanitary arrangements.
- Judy is prepared to supply a changing mat and a suitable surface to work on, as well as at least three towels.
- Judy's partner Simon, is prepared to look after Alfie if he is to be present during the delivery, or to make alternative arrangements for him.
- Judy and Simon understand the limitations of resuscitation in a home delivery setting and are aware that emergency transfer to hospital may be necessary in the case of any complications, e.g. fetal distress, and that if transfer is not possible only basic

---

resuscitation techniques of airway management and cardiac compressions will be available to their infant. Additionally, Simon must be briefed as to his course of action if he is required to contact the emergency services.

- All neonatal resuscitation equipment should be checked and in full working order.

Judy is in established labour and you are called to attend.

What are your courses of actions to prepare for the birth from the infant's perspective?

Probably, you have included the following:

- Equipment is laid out in an appropriate and convenient area. Towels are set to warm.
- Equipment is checked to be functional.
- The room is warm and draught-free, with adequate lighting.
- A clock or watch is visible to allow you to record the time taken to resuscitate the infant if necessary.
- Whilst it is not mandatory, you may choose to contact a midwife colleague to be present at the delivery.

A male infant is delivered.

What immediate parameters will you assess?

Your assessment will include the following:

- Colour
- Breathing
- Heart Rate
- Tone

He is pale and floppy, has a slow heart rate and is not breathing.

How are you going to manage this situation? Assume you have a colleague present to manage the continuing care of Judy.

Action plan

- Receive the infant into one of the warmed towels whilst under-taking your assessment. This infant has undergone some degree of compromise. He is pale with a slow heart rate, which suggests inadequate oxygenation and peripheral shutdown. He therefore needs immediately to open his airway and establish breathing.
- Note the time as this will be important in recording time to first spontaneous breath.
- Transfer him to the prepared space, dry him thoroughly, remove the wet towel, and cover his head and extremities to reduce heat loss. The chest needs to be exposed to observe for respiratory activity. Ensure that the cord is securely clamped to avoid any accidental bleeding under the towel.
- The airway must be opened and five slow sustained rescue breaths given via a 500-ml self-inflating bag attached to 100 per cent oxygen.

You undertake these manoeuvres and the chest has not moved

What is your next course of action?

Action plan

- Reassess the head position and your technique: is the infant's head overextended or flexed, impeding the airway?
- Have you got an appropriately-sized face-mask and is it held firmly, avoiding leaks?
- Check these and attempt five slow sustained rescue breaths.

The chest still does not move, despite your technique being correct.

What will you do next?

Action plan

- Consider suction; whilst there is no obvious meconium, other particulate matter may be occluding the airway.
- Being mindful of the potential adverse sequela of suction, remember that you can help avoid complications if:

→

- pressure is controlled to 100mmHg maximum;
- a large-bore catheter is used to enable removal of thick particulate matter;
- the depth of insertion is limited to no more than 5 cm from lips;
- the time of suction is limited to five seconds.

The suction reveals a thick mucoid plug. Five slow sustained inflation breaths are again attempted. This time the chest moves with each inflation.

What are you going to do now?

Action plan

- After 20–30 seconds of ventilation breaths, i.e. 15 to 20 breaths, check the heart rate for a response.
- If the heart rate less than 60bpm, commence chest compression.
- If the heart rate greater than 60 *and rising,* continue with ventilation breaths until the infant is making spontaneous breathing effort.

The infant is now two minutes of age, is making good spontaneous breathing efforts and is becoming pink, with a heart rate greater than 100 bpm. What are you going to do now?

Action plan

- Remove the face-mask from the infant's face, but continue to give some free-flow oxygen to ensure that the colour is maintained and observe his breathing pattern, heart rate and tone.
- Once he is vigorous and pink without oxygen give him to the parents and explain the sequence of events. Ensure that his temperature is maintained by undertaking skin-to-skin contact with Judy with his exposed surface and head covered, or ensure he is properly wrapped to reduce heat losses and thermal stress.

Managing Childbirth Emergencies in Community Settings

Although the situation has been managed effectively, reflect upon other action which might have been necessary:

* Insertion of a Guedel airway to stabilise airway more effectively.
* A 2–3-cm pad under his shoulders could have helped with airway patency.
* If the heart rate had not increased following chest movement, chest compression would have been indicated.
* Continued resuscitation would have triggered Simon calling for the emergency services when you instructed him to do so.

Also make a mental plan of how you would have managed this situation in the absence of a second midwife.

References

Ackermann-Liebrich U, Voegeli T, Gunter-Witt K, Kunz I, Zullig M, Schindler C and Maurer M, Zurich Study Team (1996) Home Versus Hospital Deliveries: Follow-up Study of Matched Pairs for Procedures and Outcome; _British Medical Journal_ **313**, 1313–8.

Berry P J (1992) Perinatal Postmortem. In N R C Roberton (ed), _Textbook of Neonatology_. Churchill Livingstone: London.

Björklund L J and Hellström-Westas L (2000) Reducing Heat Loss at Birth in Very Preterm Infants, _Journal of Pediatrics_ **137** (5), 739–40.

BMJ Working Party (1997) _Resuscitation of Babies at Birth_. BMJ Publishing Group: London.

Bocking A, White S E, Homan J and Richardson B S (1992) Oxygen Consumption is Maintained in Fetal Sheep During Prolonged Hypoxaemia, _Journal of Developmental Physiology_ **17**, 169–174.

Broomfield R (1996) A Quasi-Experimental Research to Investigate the Retention of Basic Cardiopulmonary Resuscitation Skills and Knowledge by Qualified Nurses Following a Course in Professional Development, _Journal of Advanced Nursing_ **23** (5), 1016–23.

Casalaz D M, Marlow N and Speidal B D (1998) Outcome of Resuscitation Following Unexpected Apparent Stillbirth, _Archives Diseases in Childhood_ **78**, F112–5.

CESDI (Confidential Enquiry into Stillbirths and Deaths in Infancy) (1995), _3rd Annual Report_. Maternal and Child Health Research Consortium: London.

CESDI (Confidential Enquiry into Stillbirths and Deaths in Infancy) (2001), _8th Annual Report_. Maternal and Child Health Research Consortium: London.

Chamberlain G, Wraight A and Crowley P (1999) Birth at Home, _Practicing Midwife_ **2** (7), 35–9.

Chameides L and Hazinski M F (1997) *Pediatric Advanced Life Support.* American Heart Association: Dallas, TX.

Cohn H E, Sacks E J Heymann, M A and Rudolph A M (1974) Cardiovascular Responses to Hypoxia and Acidaemia in Fetal Lambs; *America Journal of Obstetrics and Gynecology* **120**, 817–24.

David R (1988) Closed Chest Cardiac Massage in the Newborn Infant, *Pediatrics* **81**, 552–4.

Davies J, Hey E, Redid W and Young G (1996) Prospective Regional Study of Planned Home Births, *British Medical Journal* **313**, 1302–6.

Daze A M and Scanlon J W (1981) *Code Pink. A Practical System for Neonatal/Perinatal Resuscitation.* University Park Press: Baltimore, MD.

Donn S M (1998) *Risk Management in Neonatal Practice.* Abstract presented at 6th Annual Neonatal Conference, Middlesborough, UK.

Greenough A (1995) Meconium Aspiration Syndrome – Prevention and Treatment, *Early Human Development* **41**, 183–92.

Halliday H (1992) Other Acute Lung Disorders. In J C Sinclair and M B Bracken (eds), *Effective Care of the Newborn* Oxford University Press: Oxford.

Levene M I (1995) The Asphyxiated Newborn Infant. In M I Levene and R J Lilford (eds), *Fetal and Neonatal Neurology and Neurosurgery* (2nd edn). Churchill Livingstone: Edinburgh.

Lundstrom K E, Pryds O and Greisen G (1995) Oxygen at Birth and Prolonged Cerebral Vasoconstriction in Preterm Infants, *Archives Diseases in Childhood* **73**, F81–6.

Maternity Services Advisory Committee (1984) *Maternity Care in Action Part II Care during Childbirth (Intrapartum Care): A Guide to Good Practice and a Plan for Action.* HMSO: London.

Menegazzi J J, Auble T E, Nicklas K A, Hosack G M, Rack L and Goode J S (1993) Two Thumb Versus Two Finger Chest Compression during CPR in a Swine Infant Model of Cardiac Arrest, *Annals of Emergency Medicine* **22** (2), 112–15.

Methven R C (1993) The Antenatal Booking Interview. In J Alexander; V Levy and S Roch (eds), *Antenatal Care. A Research Based Approach.* Macmillan: London.

Milner A D (1995) Resuscitation at Birth. In M C Colquhoun A J Handley and T R Evans (eds), *ABC of Resuscitation* (3rd edn). BMJ Publishing Group: London.

NMC (Nursing and Midwifery Council) (2002) *Guidelines for Records and Record Keeping.* NMC: London.

Phibbs R H (1994) Delivery Room Management. In G B Avery, M A Fletcher and M G Macdonald (eds), *Neonatology Pathophysiology and Management of the Newborn* (4th edn) Lippencott: Philadelphia, PA.

Raivio K O (1996) Neonatal Organ Damage Due to Ischaemia Reperfusion, *Biology of the Neonate* **69**, 170–1.

Ramji S, Ahuja S, Thirupuram S, Rootwelt T, Rooth G and Saugstaad O D (1993) Resuscitation of Asphyxic Newborn Infants in Room Air or 100% Oxygen, *Pediatric Research* **34** (6), 809–12.

Rennie J (1996) Perinatal Management at the Lower Margin of Viability, *Archives of Disease in Childhood* **74**, F214–8.

Resuscitation Council (UK) (2001a) *Newborn Life Support Instructor Manual.* Resuscitation Council (UK): London.

Resuscitation Council (UK) (2001b) *Resuscitation at Birth. The Newborn Life Support Provider Course Manual.* Resuscitation Council (UK): London.

Roberton N R C (1992) Resuscitation of the Newborn. In N R C Roberton (ed), *Textbook of Neonatology* (2nd edn). Churchill Livingstone: London.

Rootwelt T, Loberg E M, Moen A, Oyasaeter S and Saugstaad O D (1992) Hypoxaemia and Reoxygenation with 21% or 100% Oxygen in Newborn Piglets: Changes in Blood Pressure, Base Deficit, and Hypoxanthine and Brain Morphology, *Pediatric Research* **32** (1), 107–13.

Royal College of Midwives (2002) Position Paper 25: Home Birth, *Royal College of Midwives Journal* **5** (1), 26–9.

Rutter N (1992) Temperature Control and its Disorders. In N R C Roberton (ed), *Textbook of Neonatology* (2nd edn). Churchill Livingstone: London.

Saugstad O D (1998a) Practical Aspects of Resuscitating Asphyxiated Newborn Infants, *European Journal of Pediatrics* **157** (Supp. 1), S11–5.

Saugstad O D (1998b) Oxygen Radical Disease in Neonatology, *Seminars in Neonatology* **3**, 231–8.

Saugstad O D, Rootwelt T and Aalen O (1998) Resuscitation of Asphyxiated Newborn Infants with Room Air or Oxygen: An International Controlled Trial: The Resair 2 Study. Electronic abstracts http://www. *Pediatrics.org.*

Sosensko I L S, Chen Y, Price L T and Lee F (1995) Failure of Premature Rabbits to Increase Lung Antioxidant Enzyme Activities After Hypoxic Exposure: Antioxidant Enzyme Gene Expression and Pharmacologic Interventions with Endotoxin and Dexamethasone, *Pediatric Research* **37** (4), 469–75.

Talner N S, Lister G and Fahey J T (1992) Effects of Asphyxia on the Myocardium of the Fetus and Newborn. In R A Polin and W W Fox (eds), *Fetal and Neonatal Physiology.* W B Saunders: Philadelphia.

UKCC (United Kingdom Central Council for Nursing, Midwifery and Health Visiting) (1998) *Midwives Rules and Code of Practice.* UKCC: London.

Vohra S, Frent G, Campbell V, Abbott M and Whyte R (1999) Effect of Polythene Occlusive Skin Wrapping on Heat Loss in Very Low Birth Weight Infants at Delivery: A Randomized Trial, *Journal of Pediatrics* **134**, 547–51.

Vyas H, Milner A D, Hopkin I E and Boon A W (1981) Physiologic Response to Prolonged and Slow – Rise Inflation in the Resuscitation of the Asphyxiated Newborn, *Journal of Pediatrics* **99**, 635–9.

Weigers T A, Keirse M J N C, van der Zee J and Berghs G A H (1996) Outcome of Planned Home and Planned Hospital Births in Low Risk Pregnancies: Prospective Study in Midwifery Practices in the Netherlands, *British Medical Journal* **313**, 1309–13.

Wiswell T E and Bent R C (1993) Meconium Staining and the Meconium Aspiration Syndrome. Unresolved Issues, *Pediatric Clinics of North America* **40** (5), 955–76.

Zander L and Chamberlain G (1999) ABC of Labour Care (Clinical Review), *British Medical Journal* **318**, 721–3.

Ziderman D A, Bingham R, Beattie T, Bland J, Bruins-Stassen M, Frei F, Gamsu H, Hamilton P, Milner A, Pepper P, Phillips B, Riesgo L, Speer C and Van Reempts P (1998) Recommendations on Resuscitation of Babies at Birth, *Resuscitation* **37**, 103–10.

8

The Paramedic's Perspective

John Scott and Natasha Taylor

Introduction

Many professional groups in the health service have numerous years of tradition and development which forms the basis of their current status and the care they provide. In contrast, up until relatively recently, attitudes and practices within the ambulance services have hardly altered. The ambulance services arose from a local authority background, providing little more than a transport service between the community and hospitals and responding only when asked. Today, changes in the service are accelerating rapidly and ambulance trusts are now very sophisticated organisations. They use deployment methods to predict service requirements and staffing levels, and provide pre-arrival telephone instructions or advice, different types of ambulance response and out-of-hospital treatments across the total range of National Health Service (NHS) provision.

The most significant change must be the increased level of knowledge and skill that the ambulance staff now possess (both ambulance technicians and paramedics), together with the equipment and drugs that they can use. Developments in the training and education of ambulance staff and the introduction of paramedic registration have had a major impact on out-of-hospital clinical practice. While still very much evolving, there is now recognition of the role that ambulance services can play in providing whole system health care, and new interprofessional partnerships are being established to provide well-integrated services.

Surprisingly, it is in the field of obstetrics that changes have been

slowest to develop and professional relationships have been more difficult to establish. Flying squads, in which an ambulance would transport
'the team' into the community and return the patient back to the hospital, are a thing of the past. Yet there is a wide deficit of knowledge about
the contemporary scope of the ambulance service, including the assistance that they are able to provide in the event of maternal collapse and
hospital transfer.

Changes in the provision of obstetric care has taken place with little
consideration of the role of the ambulance services, and it appears essential in the face of increased community-based maternity care that the
existing, rigid multiprofessional boundaries become more flexible in
order to provide a more fully integrated service for community care and
interfacility transfers.

Ambulance services are central to the management of childbirth
complications and emergencies in the community, and this chapter aims
to provide information about the education and training of and assistance provided by the ambulance technicians and paramedics in order
to promote an effective team approach to care.

Ambulance staff training in obstetrics

Babies and their delivery have never been respecters of planning or
timing and, coupled with the vagaries of adult behaviour, this has meant
that obstetric delivery and the management of both mothers and babies
has always been part of ambulance life. Indeed, it is often one of the
most harrowing and yet rewarding aspects of any ambulance professional's career when s(he) assists in the delivery of a near-term or term
baby. The other end of the spectrum is the delivery of the very premature baby, often in circumstances that are far from ideal, and this can tax
even the most competent paramedic. With these types of incidents
occurring not infrequently (in 1998, obstetric calls accounted for approximately 4 per cent of the total 999 workload), it is surprising that the
educational aspects of obstetric and neonatal care have not received
greater attention.

In reviewing the old ambulance training manuals, there is little
mention of obstetrics or neonatal management and it was not until the
publication of the *Changing Childbirth* report (DoH 1993), following on
from the recommendations in the Winterton report (House of Commons
Health Select Committee 1992) that this began to change.

Ambulance services training is funded by primary care trusts (PCTs), previously health authorities, as part of their provision of emergency ambulance services and not from Non-Medical Education and Training (NMET) funds as in the case of other health professional groups, although this may change following the introduction of Workforce Development Confederations. When the *Changing Childbirth* report recommendations were released, each health authority decided whether or not it was going to support financially any additional ambulance paramedic training. In a number of ambulance trusts some staff received the extra obstetric training and some did not. There was also variation across the country between ambulance trusts in the length of the basic training courses and in the provision of on-going continuing professional development. As a result, on an individual basis, the level of training in obstetrics was once quite variable.

However, those who have undertaken their basic technician or para-medic training in the past three or four years will have received the obstetric training. As ambulance services' training moved from the NHS Training Directorate (NHS TD) to the Institute of Health and Care Development (IHCD), the two levels of training for ambulance techni-cians and ambulance paramedics became standardised, with the green book for ambulance technicians (Ambulance Service 1998) and the blue book for ambulance paramedics (Ambulance Service 1999). In April 2001 obstetrics became formalised as part of paramedic training, although trauma management in relation to obstetrics saw a revision in the training syllabus in 1999. The basic ambulance technician training had changed in 1998.

The first move towards a more integrated provision of ambulance clin-ical care came with the publication of *Clinical Guidelines* by the Joint Royal Colleges Ambulance Liaison Committee (JRCALC 2000), which has a dedicated obstetrics/gynaecology chapter. These guidelines now form the basis for ambulance clinical provision across Britain. They have gradually been adopted by all ambulance trusts, and the next version is due for publication in 2004. Other things, such as the equipment carried and drugs available, have also changed in the past two to three years.

Paramedic registration

Before 1987, ambulance staff held a Miller qualification and were known as 'qualified ambulance persons'. While at that time a number of ambulance staff had undertaken training within the EMT (Emergency Medical Technician) programme and had become 'Intubation and Infusion' (I&I) trained, it was not until 1987 that the first staff with 'extended ambulance skills' made their appearance, receiving this award from the NHS TD. The ambulance strike during the winter of 1989–90 and the intervention of Kenneth Clarke, the Secretary of State at that time, paved the way for introducing the word paramedic (those with extended ambulance skills) and a requirement for a paramedic on every front-line ambulance. The function of the NHS TD moved to the IHCD as the awarding body, and the ambulance paramedic award became formally recognised. The IHCD award is the licence to practice, and those who hold this award are able to practise extended skills and to use a wider range of drugs in emergency situations.

Towards the end of the 1990s the term paramedic was used by a number of people who did not have the IHCD award. In 2000, paramedics became a professional group, and those who registered with the Committee for the Professions Supplementary to Medicine (CPSM) became State Registered Paramedics. The authority invested in the CPSM moved to the Health Professions Council (HPC) and in April 2003 the term paramedic became a title restricted to those registered with the HPC.

The paramedic profession is very much in its infancy and has still to create an effective professional body which could eventually be responsible for the educational standards for paramedics.

Although ambulance paramedics have gained the recognition they deserve, unfortunately ambulance technicians are not included in the present arrangements.

Career progression and present roles

It is essential to have a clear understanding of the terminology used and the different roles of staff in the ambulance services. When new staff (minimum age 21) join an ambulance trust, they undergo basic technician and driver training to become student ambulance technicians (SATs) for a year, before gaining their IHCD ambulance technician award to become qualified ambulance technicians (ATs). During their first year SATs should work with an experienced member of the front-line staff.

Ambulance technicians, although qualified, are limited in the number of drugs they may use and the types of invasive procedures which they can practise. Technicians may then apply to join a paramedic training course and, if successful, will undergo a period of classroom work followed by in-hospital training before completing their ambulance paramedic award and being able to apply for paramedic registration with the HPC.

Some ambulance trusts have created academic programmes, and those progressing from ambulance technician to paramedic may gain a Certificate in Higher Education. Paramedics may also progress to a Diploma in Higher Education (paramedic science), a two-year part-time course aimed at linking practical knowledge with underpinning theoretical work.

Starting in 2003, school leavers (age 18) may undertake a foundation degree and, after three years' combined academic study and work in an ambulance environment, where they will complete both the technician and paramedic awards, they will be awarded a foundation degree. All of these pathways offer the individuals academic credits which they can use to combine with further university courses in order ultimately to gain a full degree.

Within a growing number of ambulance trusts, paramedics are taking on new roles working as single responders purely within the range of ambulance responses. In the remaining trusts, paramedics are linked directly to primary care, working in general practices while still responding to ambulance emergency calls.

The most recent development has come from the Changing Workforce Programme which is leading an initiative to develop 'emergency care practitioners'. While these programmes are open to any registered health care professional, it is ambulance paramedics who are at the forefront of this development. As the new GP contract refashions the whole primary care provision, individuals undertaking these courses will be able to work in a number of primary care settings, including walk-in centres, urgent-care centres or out-of-hours systems.

The difference between ambulance technicians and paramedics

Ambulance technicians are able to undertake patient assessments and to provide many emergency life-saving treatments, particularly those linked to cardiac arrest, acute asthma, anaphylaxis and external haemorrhage.

The treatments which they can provide include oxygen therapy, defibrillation, simple airway procedures, possibly using a laryngeal mask airway or nasal airway, pain relief using Entonox®, and a number of splints such as cervical collars, traction splints and long boards.

Although ambulance paramedics may not treat a greater range of conditions, they do have a deeper understanding of the underlying clinical problems and pathophysiology. They also have a wider range of invasive procedures, including airway skills such as endotracheal intubation and jet insufflation, and may gain intravenous or intraosseous access. The range of drugs which they can use is greater, including cardiac arrest drugs, treatments for asthma, Nubain and Morphine for pain, Naloxone, and for obstetric use, Syntometrine, although few services carry this drug routinely. Additionally they can use Benzyl Penicillin for meningitis and Frusemide for the treatment of congestive heart failure, as well as thrombolytics. In addition to these drugs, a number of ambulance trusts have a range of drugs available under patient group directions for use by selected paramedics.

Calls for ambulance assistance

An aspect of ambulance activity, of which an understanding is also required, is the way in which ambulance services respond to calls for assistance. Any member of the public or a health professional may request an ambulance by dialling 999 but only certain health professionals can request that a patient be taken to hospital using the 'urgent' system (midwives being such a professional group). There are very strict but somewhat arbitrary time targets set down on the way in which ambulance services should respond to the various calls.

Urgent calls require the patient to be in the hospital within 15 minutes of the time agreed (between the professional caller and the ambulance trust) in 95 per cent of cases. However, many PCT commissioning groups only fund the ambulance service to achieve a lower response, ranging from 75 per cent to 85 per cent.

Emergency (999) calls are subdivided into a number of categories and here the target is to have an ambulance response at the patient in 8 minutes for category A calls (life-threatening calls) and, for other categories, in 14 minutes for urban ambulance trusts and 19 minutes for rural trusts.

The 8-minute response for category A calls requires the arrival of someone equipped with a defibrillator and capable in its use, be that an ambulance responder or another suitably trained person. The 14- or 19-minute response has to be with a vehicle capable of transporting a patient. The target for these two groups of calls is 75 per cent of category A calls reached in 8 minutes, while all calls have to receive an ambulance in 95 per cent of cases in either 14 or 19 minutes (DoH 1996). These targets form part of the star rating for ambulance trusts.

The ambulance response to an obstetric-related call

This section traces what happens when there is an obstetric call or potential obstetric call in the community.

The caller will dial 999 and will be asked to give ambulance control the geographic location and demographic details. They will be asked for a description of the main complaint and from this the ambulance call-taker will use a computer-driven system to question the caller to obtain certain key details about the patient. There are two systems used in Britain, both with a common end point which classifies the call and determines the speed of ambulance response required. The two systems are the Medical Priority Dispatch System (MPDS) and Criteria-Based Dispatch (CPD), and details can be obtained from your local ambulance control.

For obstetric calls, some ambulance control rooms will dispatch their own response and then may have agreements with their local obstetric units to call a community midwife or to inform the local delivery suite. In all trusts using community or first-response systems to provide early community intervention before the arrival of the ambulance response, obstetric calls are excluded.

Depending upon the type of problem and the degree of emergency, the call-taker may provide pre-arrival instructions or guidance to the caller. Indeed, callers have been guided through a rapidly advancing delivery to assist the mother before any emergency service response arrives on the scene.

The ambulance dispatcher will send the nearest available ambulance response, possibly a single responder, but will also send a fully manned and equipped ambulance. Depending upon the geographic setting, the ambulance dispatcher may be able to call upon local GPs or immediate care doctors to assist.

Certain social or religious groups require female attention during labour and birth. This presents practical problems for the ambulance services, as the majority of ambulance front-line staff are male.

The JRCALC (Joint Royal Colleges Ambulance Liaison Committee) national clinical guidelines on obstetric calls

The full set of national clinical guidelines used by ambulance trusts can be found on the JRCALC web site (www.jrcalc.org.uk) which can be accessed through the NHS net.

The JRCALC *Clinical Guidelines* chapter on obstetrics has sections on normal pregnancy, normal deliveries, abnormal deliveries including postpartum haemorrhage, eclampsia, haemorrhage during pregnancy, and sexual assault.

The overriding principles which run through these sections are to:

- consider the possibility of pregnancy in emergency situations with a wide understanding of the age range for females to be pregnant;
- be alert to the effect that the physiological changes occurring during pregnancy may have in emergency situations;
- ensure early and adequate resuscitation of the mother as the best and most effective way of supporting the fetus;
- obtain midwifery guidance urgently when dealing with a potential or imminent birth;
- be competent in adult resuscitation;
- be competent in neonatal resuscitation using the Resuscitation Council (UK) guidelines (www.resus.org.uk);

but not to:

- delay the patient transfer in the case of any obstetric abnormality or time-critical emergency if midwifery guidance is not immediately available but to proceed to the nearest obstetric unit (or A&E department) as rapidly as possible, providing an alerting message to the hospital;
- undertake specific interventional assessments or treatments related to the pregnancy.

Specific areas of care

Normal pregnancy and delivery

While obstetric units will give mothers-to-be and their partners considerable support and guidance about when to contact the delivery suite and when to make their own way to the unit once labour has started, it is not uncommon for ambulance control to receive calls to provide transport for those in labour to hospital from the community. Sometimes these calls can be in situations where the labour has advanced more quickly than was expected and the birth is imminent.

The ambulance control will dispatch an ambulance and, if possible, inform the local delivery suite. In these situations both technicians and paramedics will follow the same approach, assessing the situation and undertaking a general examination that should include pulse and blood pressure checks as well as an external examination of the abdomen and inspection of the perineum if appropriate (when the birth is imminent).

If the situation occurs in a public place then the mother will be moved rapidly to the hospital. Depending upon local agreements, this may be to the A&E department or to the delivery suite.

If pain relief is required, both technicians and paramedics can administer Entonox®. Other drugs are not advised. All ambulance staff have been taught about the consequences of vena caval compression and will position the patient accordingly. However, within reason, patients are encouraged to assume a position that is comfortable for them.

During a normal birth, ambulance staff are taught to control the descent of the baby's head but not to interfere with the progression of birth. Following the birth, the baby should be wrapped in warm towelling and given to the mother. The third stage is then allowed to progress naturally without any active intervention.

There is always a debate about cutting the cord and when that should occur. Practice varies but both technicians and paramedics are taught that if they have to separate mother and baby for clinical or practical purposes then the cord should be cut between two clamps.

Although Syntometrine is a drug available for paramedic use, the indications for which it can be used are tightly controlled. Paramedics may **not** use it during the third stage as part of active placental delivery.

Abnormal delivery

The JRCALC clinical guidelines are very clear on this subject and state:

> The following guideline is intended to provide information and guidance for paramedics. The management of abnormal deliveries should normally be undertaken by the obstetrician and the experienced midwife. In all cases of actual or suspected abnormal delivery, **LOAD and GO** must be the primary aim to assure wherever possible the best and safest outcome for mother and baby. However, on the rare occasions where the patient cannot be immediately removed advice must be sought from the local Obstetric Unit.

Whilst the guidelines explain some of the features of abnormal presentations, the message for ambulance staff is clear. The mother should be moved swiftly to the nearest hospital with an obstetric department. Basic treatment during the transfer is to include oxygen therapy or Entonox and intravenous (IV) access and correct positioning of the mother to avoid supine hypotension. The hospital must be forewarned.

If the umbilical cord appears ahead of any other presenting part, ambulance staff are advised to cover the cord with a warm saline dressing if possible or to place the cord in the vagina with minimal handling of the cord. They must set off as quickly as possible to the nearest hospital, pre-alerting the hospital and not waiting for any form of community support from either a midwife or doctor. Where appropriate, the mother should be transported on her side with some padding placed under her hips to try and raise the pelvis to take any pressure off the cord.

Eclampsia

Within the training syllabus, ambulance technicians and paramedics learn about eclampsia and the guidelines identify that fits associated with pregnancy after 20 weeks and the first day or so after delivery should be considered eclamptic since they are only very rarely due to epilepsy.

Ambulance staff are taught to recognise an eclamptic fit as a time-critical emergency and the mother must be moved to the nearest main hospital as quickly as possible, forewarning the hospital. Ambulance technicians will administer oxygen while paramedics may additionally gain IV access and either use diazemules or rectal diazepam to control the fit. (As identified in Chapter 3 on pre-eclampsia, emergency medication for fulminating pre-eclampsia/eclampsia in the community remains controversial and local guidelines should be followed.)

Haemorrhage during pregnancy

The JRCALC clinical guidelines categorise bleeding into antepartum and postpartum, with a further subdivision in antepartum bleeding being made using the twentieth week of the pregnancy as an arbitrary dividing point in time.

From the ambulance point of view, the patient assessment should proceed along the classic approach of brief history, primary survey and then secondary survey. If a time-critical feature is found, then immediate treatment and rapid transport to a hospital should take place.

Postpartum bleeding is described as being a time-critical emergency, and guidelines recommend that the patient must be moved to hospital as soon as possible and while en route to the hospital gentle massage of the uterus through the abdominal wall may be tried in an attempt to stimulate a contraction. If the bleeding is severe and the ambulance trust has trained its paramedics to use Syntometrine, then 1 ml may be given so long as the bleeding is within 24 hours of childbirth. Syntometrine may only be used by ambulance paramedics for postpartum bleeding.

Generic principles of ambulance assessments

While the guidelines give an insight into some of the particular problems that can be faced in the community when presented with someone who is pregnant, the overriding approach is that of a standard approach to any emergency call, whether the responding member of staff is an ambulance technician or paramedic.

These are:

- The principles of safety apply.
- Where appropriate, always obtain consent.
- Obtain a brief history of the event.
- Undertake a primary survey: the ABCD (airway with cervical spine protection, breathing, circulation, disability).
- Provide primary treatment – if any abnormality is found during the primary survey, this should be corrected with a move to hospital if a time-critical emergency is identified.

- Take a further and more detailed history.
- Undertake a secondary survey, including the checking of a blood glucose.
- Provide secondary treatments.
- Transfer, if appropriate.
- If remaining at the home, who should be informed?

Principles of ambulance treatments in obstetrics cases

Primary treatments

The condition is managed according to the need identified: for example correction of airway problems with or without adjuncts (endotracheal intubation is a paramedic skill); provision of oxygen and assisted ventilation; stopping of any external blood loss, defibrillation with the full range of cardiac arrest drugs, and intravenous access with fluid replacement, without delaying the progress to hospital (paramedics only).

There will be occasions when the baby requires resuscitation. Ambulance staff are taught how to recognise a sick child but have little experience with neonates. They will wrap the baby up, provide oxygen to stimulate the baby and, if more advance resuscitation is required, will follow the resuscitation guidelines.

Secondary treatments

These might include the use of splints if trauma has occurred and the use of additional drugs by paramedics. In the case of pregnancy, if a low blood glucose is found then 10 per cent glucose solutions are used.

Trauma management

Major or significant trauma in someone who happens to be pregnant does not present a management problem. The ambulance staff will take the patient to the nearest A&E department. However, there are many occasions when those who are pregnant are involved in what may superficially appear to be a minor incident. Ambulance teaching suggests that if the pregnancy is in the second or third trimester that the mother and fetus should be assessed in an obstetric unit.

Future considerations

As mentioned at the beginning of this chapter, there is scope to improve the working partnerships between midwives, obstetricians, paediatricians, general practitioners and ambulance trusts in order to provide safe community obstetric treatment coupled with an interfacility transfer system. Professional integration could be achieved relatively easily and without massive change in clinical practice. The change should be focused mainly around improved communication and understanding, and might include the following principles:

Ambulance trusts would need to ensure that following the dispatch of the ambulance response to an obstetric call, the local delivery suite or community midwifery service is alerted.

Ambulance staff would require more insight and a greater understanding of obstetric practice. This is not necessarily to enable them to undertake a different role but so that they would be able to communicate more precisely with midwives and the primary health care team during both the in-hours' and increasing out-of-hours' provision.

There would be standardisation of skills, equipment and treatments across all groups working in the community including midwives and ambulance staff and this would be supported by the PCTs.

Every group would have a clear understanding of the roles and abilities of the other groups, including the different rankings within organisations.

There would be a definite audit programme to support the provision of community obstetrics and joint meetings would become an accepted part of practice, informing and offering a forum for self-reflection and critical debriefing.

There would be discussion to understand the impact of the new GP contract on community obstetric provision and the role of ambulance trusts would be considered in any such discussions.

References

Ambulance Service (1998) *Basic Training*. Ambulance Service Association Institute of Health and Care Development (IHCD): London.

Ambulance Service (1999) *Paramedic Training*. Ambulance Service Association Institute of Health and Care Development (IHCD): London.

DoH (Department of Health) (1993) *Changing Childbirth. The Report of the Expert Maternity Group. Part One*. HMSO: London.

DoH (Department of Health) (1996) *Review of Ambulance Performance Standards. Final Report of Steering Group*, July. HMSO: London.

House of Commons Health Select Committee (1992) *Second Report on the Maternity Services* (Chairman Mr N Winterton). HMSO: London.

JRCALC (Joint Royal Colleges Ambulance Liaison Committee) (2000) *Clinical Guidelines*, www.jrcalc.org.uk

9

Risk Management and Other Legal Considerations

Amanda Williamson and Kenda Crozier

Introduction

As identified in Chapter 1, midwives have accepted immense responsibility in developing community-based midwifery services and fulfilling the essential prerequisite of being adequately prepared to manage unanticipated childbirth emergencies in the absence of medical support. This chapter aims to support midwives in their goal of increasing women's childbirth options by exploring a number of important professional and legal issues. It will begin with a discussion of clinical governance and the identification of risk management activities. The chapter will then go on to address professional and legal accountability, including issues of consent and refusal of treatment, and the principles of how midwives can practise safely and competently within the boundaries of their professional and legal framework. Finally, the legal position regarding the right to a home birth is explored.

Clinical governance and risk management

Clinical governance is:

> A framework through which NHS (National Health Service) organisations are accountable for continuously improving the quality of their services and

safeguarding high standards of care by creating an environment in which excellence in clinical care will flourish. (DoH 1998 p. 33)

The process of clinical governance involves a number of activities in which risk management plays a pivotal role and applies to everyone who provides or manages patient or client care and services. Other areas, which make up the framework of clinical governance, include continuing professional education, statutory supervision, multidisciplinary working, evidence-based practice, user involvement, clinical audit, and standard setting. Midwives already use many of these tools within their practice. Clinical governance falls under the umbrella of the National Institute for Clinical Excellence (NICE). This organisation promotes clinical effectiveness and cost-efficient services for NHS patients by providing guidelines for best practice based on sound evidence. As yet there are no national guidelines for midwives undertaking home deliveries, although the Secretary of State for Health announced in February 2003 that a review of maternity services will be undertaken to ensure national standards for all aspects of maternity care. For any midwife practising in the home care setting, these national standards (once agreed) will be a valuable guide to the expected standard of practice.

The most important area of clinical governance to be considered within the context of emergency situations may well be risk management. The Royal College of Obstetricians and Gynaecologists (RCOG 2001 p. 1) defines clinical risk management as:

> methods for the early identification of adverse events using either staff reports or systematic screening of records. This should be followed by a creation of a database to identify common patterns and develop a system of accountability to prevent future incidents.

This definition highlights the importance of risk management as a tool to improve quality of care rather than to minimise litigation. Since it is there to improve patient and client care, it is therefore clear that the responsibility for risk management lies with individual practitioners as well as with organisations. Mills and von Bolschwing (1995) assert that any effective risk management system needs to start with an accurate assessment of the risks. Obviously, although an emergency may be sudden and unforeseen, it is important that midwives be able to analyse and understand the risks involved whilst providing care in the community. The midwife has an opportunity to undertake risk assessment of all clients at initial booking and this provides valuable information to help minimise adverse outcomes later in the pregnancy. The risk assessment made at initial booking should be acted upon and, rather than being a one-off event, needs continually to be re-evaluated throughout care. Williams (1995 p. 175) claims that 'A more proactive approach to case management will not only provide higher quality care, it will also control the risks, thus reducing the likelihood of adverse outcomes.'

A further way in which risks may be identified is by examining critical incidents retrospectively and particularly those with unexpected outcomes (NICE 2001). The Confidential Enquiry into Stillbirths and Deaths in Infancy (CESDI) and the Confidential Enquiry into Maternal Deaths (CEMD) provide guidelines for effective management of care by analysing cases in which something has gone wrong. These now come under the auspices of the Confidential Enquiries into Maternal and Child Health (CEMACH). These enquiries give midwives valuable advice when dealing with adverse situations within both hospital and home settings. For example, in the most recent Confidential Enquiry into Maternal Deaths (NICE 2001) there is a chapter dedicated to midwifery practice recommendations. There are also recommendations for practice within CESDI reports. Any midwife in practice (particularly those practising away from an obstetric-led unit) should be aware of, and if possible follow, the recommendations from these enquiries.

National Health Service (NHS) Trusts must set standards for care based on risk assessment and these often incorporate recommendations from the reports of CESDI and CEMD. The policies and guidelines should provide a standard set of evidence-based protocols that cover all areas in which care may be provided, including the home, clinics and hospitals. Midwives should be familiar with both the recommendations of CEMACH and their employer's policies and practice guidelines. However, midwives should always ensure that they practise within the scope of practice, whilst acknowledging their own limitations (UKCC 1998). The employer's guidelines and protocols may not always seem appropriate in an emergency setting away from the hospital environment. Where no policy applies, then the midwife must rely upon her own knowledge and clinical judgement, and practise safely within the Midwives Rules and Code of Practice (UKCC 1998) and the Code of Professional Conduct (NMC 2002a). Kennedy (1993) observes that guidelines are increasingly being used to judge the standard of care provided by doctors in the law and the same must surely be true of any professional working within the NHS, including midwives.

Clinical governance requires that all clinical practice be evidence-based and the Nursing and Midwifery Council (NMC) states: '[As a registered midwife] you have a responsibility to deliver care based on current evidence, best practice and, where applicable, validated research when it is available' (NMC 2002a p. 8).

In order to practise effectively and proficiently the NMC (2002a) requires that practitioners regularly undertake activities to update their knowledge and skills, and practise within their sphere of competence.

Rule 40 of the Midwives Rules states:

> Except in an emergency, a practising midwife shall not provide any midwifery care or undertake any treatment which she has not, either before or after registration as a midwife, been trained to give or which is outside her current sphere of practice. (UKCC 1998 p. 17)

When midwives undertake responsibility for a client they must ensure that they are qualified to administer safe and effective care, whilst also acknowledging their own limitations of practice.

In the emergency situation a midwife would reasonably be expected to call for help or assistance from an appropriately qualified professional. In the case of an emergency in the home, this may be a general practitioner, a paramedic or another midwife. The Royal College of Obstetricians and Gynaecologists and Royal College of Midwives (RCOG/RCM 1999) recommend that all maternity care staff should receive regular training and updating on the management of emergency situations. The Clinical Negligence Scheme for Trusts (CNST 2002) also incorporates this recommendation in its standards for clinical risk management for the maternity services. Many maternity units incorporate these recommendations into the post-registration education provision for midwives, and it would be advisable for all midwives to access this valuable resource in order that they have experience of simulated emergency situations.

If a midwife is in the unfortunate position of being in an emergency situation away from an obstetric-led unit, the supervisor of midwives should be informed as soon as possible so that the midwife may receive appropriate advice and support (UKCC 1998).

Professional and legal accountability

Professional accountability

Midwives may be held accountable for their practice either by their professional body, the NMC, or by the law. There are a number of definitions of accountability. Perhaps one of the best is that of Murray and Zentner (1989, p. 88): 'being responsible for one's acts and being able to explain, define or measure in some way the results of decision making'. This makes it imperative that midwives accept responsibility and are able to provide a sound rationale for their practice. Midwives must also demonstrate that the care given was safe and effective, thus evaluating the outcomes of their care.

The Midwives Rules and Code of Practice (UKCC 1998) defines the scope of acceptable midwifery practice within the law. Rule 40 identifies that a practising midwife has responsibility for providing care for women and their infants in the antepartum, intrapartum and postpartum periods. The NMC Code of Professional Conduct (2002a para. 1:3) states:

> You are personally accountable for your practice. This means that you are answerable for your actions and omissions regardless of advice or directions from another professional.

Despite the stress of an emergency situation and possible pressure to step outside statutory professional boundaries, it is particularly important to adhere to the Midwives Rules and Code of Practice and Code of Professional Conduct. This will help midwives protect themselves from allegations of misconduct and litigation.

The NMC will consider any complaints of professional misconduct made by fellow midwives, other professionals, and clients and their families or employers. In 2000, 22 per cent of all complaints made against professionals on the UKCC register came from members of the public (UKCC 2000). The NMC can only consider complaints which are potentially serious enough to lead to removal of a practitioner's name from the register. The NMC (2002b p. 3) states: 'The purpose of our proceedings is to protect the public, rather than to punish nurses and midwives.'

If a complaint is received by the NMC, it examines the case, takes statements and forwards all the evidence to the Preliminary Proceedings Committee (PPC) for consideration. The PPC proceedings are private in order to protect the identity of the practitioner. At this point, the case can either be closed or forwarded to a full public hearing, or a caution can be issued which will remain on record for five years. The practitioner may be subject to an interim suspension if it is felt that there is a high risk to the public if the individual is allowed to continue in practice. The Professional Conduct Committee then hears the case. Under the UKCC the facts of the case needed to be proven 'beyond reasonable doubt'. This is the same high standard of proof required as that for a criminal court. However, the NMC is bringing about changes in the way in which professional conduct cases are dealt with, including the burden of proof standard (NMC 2003). In future the standard will be the lesser standard required under civil law: the defendant need only prove the case on the 'balance of probabilities'. If a practitioner is found guilty of professional misconduct, the PCC has a number of options which include removing the practitioner's name from the register.

It is important, therefore, when dealing with an emergency situation that midwives act within the boundaries of midwifery practice (UKCC 1998) and within trust guidelines wherever possible, and that they seek appropriate assistance. In doing so, they are safeguarding their own practice as well as protecting women.

Legal accountability

Midwives are accountable in law for their actions and omissions. Depending upon the complaint made against them, the legal proceedings initiated may be under criminal or civil law.

Civil law

The majority of medical cases initiated are generally civil or tort. A tort concerns disputes between individuals and the state steps in as an intermediary to settle the dispute. The reasons that most proceedings are civil may well be the lower standard of proof required (the balance of probabilities) and the possible payment of damages. In criminal law (mentioned later) there is a higher standard of proof required (beyond reasonable doubt) and monetary reward in the form of criminal compensation is lower.

Obstetrics is a key area for negligence claims (CNST 2002). To prove a negligent action the following criteria must be met: first it must be proved that the professional owed the claimant a duty of care; secondly it must be established that the duty of care was breached; thirdly it must be proved that the harm was caused by the breach of the duty of care and that the harm was reasonably foreseeable as a result of that breach. It is only when all conditions have been proven that damages may be assessed and awarded.

Duty of care

Legally there is little doubt that a midwife in practice owes a duty of care to her clients: 'You have a duty of care to your patients and clients, who are entitled to receive safe and competent care ' (NMC 2002a p. 3).

The definition of duty of care in law was established in Donoghue v. Stevenson (1932 AC562 at 580). It states: 'You must take reasonable care to avoid acts or omissions which you can reasonably foresee would be likely to injure your neighbour'; that 'persons who are so closely and directly affected by my act that I ought reasonably have them in contemplation as being so affected when I am directing my mind to the acts or omissions which are called in question'.

For midwives in practice, any client will be 'closely and directly' affected by their acts or omissions. In an emergency situation possibly even more so.

Breaching duty of care

In order to avoid breaching their duty of care, midwives must practise to the standard of the ordinary midwife. The test for the expected standard of care is known as the Bolam Test. It is the principle applied to all professionals. It was first articulated in Bolam v. Friern Hospital Management Committee (1957 p. 121) McNair said:

> The test is the standard of the ordinary skilled man exercising and professing to have that special skill. A man need not possess the highest expert skill at the risk of being found negligent. It is well-established law that it is sufficient if he exercises the ordinary skill of an ordinary competent man exercising that particular art.

The courts will ascertain the standard of care based upon accepted midwifery practice as it existed at the time. This means that midwives are judged according to the prevailing standard of their peers at the time that the incident took place. That is, if the incident occurred ten years ago the standard would be the accepted practice at that time. The court may well look to the Code of Professional Conduct and the Midwives Rules and Code of Practice existing at the time, as well as other midwifery and obstetric opinion, to ascertain prevailing standards of midwifery care. This underlines the importance of practising to the agreed standard of national guidelines and trust protocols as well as that of the NMC. However, the current climate of fear of litigation within the NHS has led to a vast array of regulations and guidelines being developed within individual trusts. According to Hurwitz (1995), it could be argued that these documents are a means of controlling the behaviour of medical and other staff within institutions and can interfere with a clinician's right to use his or her professional judgement in practice. He asks: 'Could compliance with guidelines protect health care workers from liability?' The fact that guidelines exist may not mean that they are a true representation of customary practice, and that is the test which will be applied in law. Thus a midwife must be able to justify any clinical decision she makes, particularly in an emergency situation away from the obstetric-led unit where there may be no guidelines available.

The Bolam Test has been accepted by the House of Lords as the expected standard of practice in relation to diagnosis (Maynard v. West Midlands Regional Health Authority 1985). An ordinary midwife could reasonably be expected to diagnose a breech presentation, for example, and institute reasonable measures to deal with the situation. In delivering treatment, Bolam is also the expected standard, but not all medical mistakes are negligent. In Whitehouse v. Jordan (1980 p. 658) the Master of the Rolls said:

> In a professional man, an error of judgement is not negligent. To test this I would suggest that you ask the average competent and careful practitioner: is this the sort of mistake that you yourself might have made? If he says 'yes even doing the best I could, it could have happened to me' then it is not negligent.

The law, therefore, affords some protection in that midwives are required to work to the standard of their peers rather than an expert practitioner. Expert witnesses called by either legal side will offer a professional opinion on whether or not the practitioner was working to the acceptable standards of the day.

Did the breach in the duty of care cause the harm?

In order to prove causation, a client must show a causal link between the breach of care and the harm that occurred. That is to say that the client must show that but for the defendant's negligence, the harm would not have occurred. In the case of Wilsher v. Essex Area Health Authority (1988), it was held that the injury could have been attributable to a number of different agents. Therefore, causation was not proven. This means that a midwife can only be held responsible if it can be proven that the midwife's negligent action caused the harm.

Even if a woman making a complaint against a midwife can prove there was a breach of the duty of care, therefore, she must also prove that the harm was caused by the actions of the midwife and that the harm was foreseeable.

Criminal law and liability

The midwife could also be held to account under criminal law. Gross negligence on behalf of a professional leading to death may lead to a conviction for manslaughter. The test was established in R v. Batemen (1925 p. 12) in which it was stated: 'The negligence of the accused went beyond a mere matter of compensation between subjects and showed such a disregard for the life and safety of others as to amount to a crime against the state and conduct deserving punishment.'

The law has further been clarified in R v. Adomako (1995 p. 178). In this case the House of Lords held that the defendant was properly convicted of involuntary manslaughter if:

> The ordinary principles of the law of negligence apply to ascertain whether or not the defendant has been in breach of a duty of care towards the victim who has died. If such breach of duty is established the next question is whether that breach of duty caused the death of the victim. If so, the jury must go on to consider whether that breach of duty should be characterised as gross negligence and therefore as a crime.

It will be considered a crime if 'Having regard to the risk of death involved, the conduct of the defendant was so bad in all the circumstances as to amount in their [the jury's] judgement to a criminal act or omission.'

Any midwife who had been responsible for a case in which her actions might have led to the death of a mother or baby could face criminal proceedings if she were found guilty of the above test. The jury would need to find that she was guilty of gross negligence 'beyond reasonable doubt'. These cases are obviously extremely rare and safe practitioners who practise within the Midwives Rules and Code of Practice (UKCC 1998) and Code of Professional Conduct (NMC 2002a) very unlikely to find themselves in this situation.

Limitation and record-keeping

The Limitation Act 1980 allows that an action must be brought within three years of the infliction of the injury or from the time of knowledge of the injury. However, if the harm is to a fetus or neonate then the three-year period can start from the time they reach majority. Under Sections 11 and 14 of the Act, if a person is unaware of the injury or did not know that negligence might have caused the injury, then the three-year period starts from the date they did or by which they should reasonably have discovered the facts. Section 33 allows the court to overrule the three-year period if it is inequitable to do so. It is essential, therefore, that midwifery and obstetric records, diaries and other papers relating to clients be kept in excess of 21 years, and storage of these can be arranged by the local trust. A midwife can still be called to account for cases in which she was involved a long time previously, and good record-keeping is, therefore, essential.

When keeping records of care episodes the midwife should demonstrate a sound rationale for decisions and actions. Clearly in an emergency situation it may not be possible for the midwife to keep contemporaneous records as required by the Midwives Rules and Code of Practice (UKCC 1998) and in this situation it is necessary to write retrospective notes as soon as is reasonably practical. All records should be written legibly and all entries should be dated and timed using the 24-hour clock and kept in a chronological order. It is important to record at what time assistance was called, the name of the person called (not just 'doctor') and the time he or she arrived. Unapproved abbreviations and the use of ambiguous terms should be avoided. The client's name and hospital number, if available, should be clearly marked on each sheet. There should be a precise record of vital signs recordings and if these were not undertaken the midwife should document why. Timings of any procedures and drugs given need to be accurately recorded. Appreciating that this is an emergency situation, the midwife should, if possible, try to write down brief comments and the times of key events which will later help form the basis of full and accurate notes. These notes are important not only as a record of an emergency situation but also because they may be used for clinical audit. They may also form crucial evidence of any litigation claim or professional misconduct case and are an opportunity for the midwife to account for her actions.

Consent and informed choice

In any emergency situation, consent will be an important consideration. Legal consent was defined in Schloendorff v. Society of NY Hospital (1914): 'Every human being of adult years and sound mind has a right to determine what shall be done with his own body; and a surgeon who performs an operation without the person's consent commits an assault.'

Consent may be implied. For example, if a midwife says to a woman, 'I would like to take your blood pressure', by holding out her arm, the woman implies her consent. Consent may be expressly obtained in writing or verbally. Written consent should, if possible, be obtained for any invasive procedure. Consent must be obtained from the person who is to receive the care. However, the adult must be competent to give the consent. This means that they must be able to appreciate what will be done to them and understand the likely consequences of leaving the condition untreated. In certain circumstances, care may be given without a person's consent and this would include an emergency situation where a person was unable to consent for himself/herself.

In regard to consent for treatment, the NMC (2002a) clearly states that consent for treatment or care must be obtained after the patient or client has received information. However Section 3.2 describes the right of the client to refuse treatment:

> You must respect patients' and clients' autonomy – their right to decide whether or not to undergo any health care intervention – even where a refusal may result in harm or death to themselves or a foetus, unless a court of law orders to the contrary. This right is protected in law, although in circumstances where the health of the foetus would be severely compromised by any refusal to give consent, it would be appropriate to discuss this matter fully within the team, and possibly to seek external advice and guidance. (NMC 2002a p. 4)

In giving information to women and obtaining consent for treatment or procedures, therefore, the midwife must make the client aware of *all foreseeable risks* involved in the course of action that she has chosen. Consequently, if a woman at risk of postpartum haemorrhage, in the light of past medical history, requests a home birth, the midwife has a duty to give the woman all available information to enable her to make a decision about care. If the midwife fails to inform her of the risks involved in choosing to have her baby at home, the midwife may be held accountable. The test of liability in relation to warning patients of risks associated to care was established in Sidaway v. Bethlem RHG (1985 p.

643) where it was stated that 'The doctor was required to act in accordance with a practice accepted at the time as proper by a responsible body of medical opinion.' It goes on to state that 'The disclosure of a particular risk of serious adverse consequences might be so obviously necessary for the patient to make an informed choice that no prudent doctor would fail to disclose that risk.'

It is, therefore, vital that the midwife explains all risks and consequences to the client so that the woman may make an informed choice and the discussion of risks should be documented. Although the *Changing Childbirth* report (DoH 1993) advocated the right of a woman to choose, this does not mean that midwives can abdicate the responsibility to give advice and information on the choices made by the woman. In fact, a midwife would breach her duty of care if she were not to give a woman a frank professional opinion using sound evidence-based information. The midwife must act in a reasonable and responsible manner because her actions may be subject to scrutiny and she needs to account for decisions made and actions taken.

The right of a mother to determine her own autonomy cannot be overruled because she is pregnant, even if her own life or that of the fetus is at risk. This was established in St George's Health Care NHS Trust v. S (1998 p. 728) where it was stated that 'A pregnant woman was entitled, as an adult of sound mind, to refuse medical treatment, even if her own life and that of the unborn child depended upon such treatment.'

If, in her professional opinion, the midwife considers that the woman is making an unsafe choice, for example in requesting a home birth when she has a history of serious postpartum haemorrhage, the midwife can seek advice from her supervisor of midwives. The supervisor may agree to see the woman and the midwife together and have a further discussion about the risks involved. It might be possible to offer some adaptation to the hospital environment that would make the option of a hospital birth acceptable to the woman. If the woman still intends to continue with her plans for a home birth, it is important to maintain good lines of communication with her to ensure that care can be provided in an emergency. The midwife should continue to provide care for the woman and draw up an action plan in collaboration with the supervisor of midwives to ensure that all risks are minimised and that contingency plans are in place to deal with any untoward incidents. The RCM (2002 p. 4) suggests that a plan should include the following:

- The woman should be adequately informed of the possible risks and their consequences.
- Two skilled and experienced midwives should be available to provide the necessary care.
- There should be liaison with the obstetric and paediatric teams to ensure that appropriate back-up is in place.
- Practice drills should be undertaken for any relevant emergency procedures.
- Professional and personal support should be available to help the midwife with any anxiety or distress she may experience.

In essence there is no reason why a midwife's duty of care should be greater towards women birthing in hospital than towards women birthing at home.

Their right to a home birth

The law in the UK does not insist that women should attend hospital for the birth of their baby but health authorities are obliged to provide a maternity service, though provision for home birth is not made explicit (RCM 2002). However, this does not give women an inalienable right to give birth at home, because the law does not provide for a home birth service to be in place in all areas.

Health service users do not have the right to insist that a particular treatment be available in their area. If it could be shown that the treatment were cost-effective and a sound use of resources, then it would be difficult to argue against the case for a home birth (Dimond 2002). As yet the law in relation to home birth has not been tested. A request for a judicial review of a case where a home birth had been refused by an NHS trust would provide clarification of the law in this area.

However, the *Changing Childbirth* Report (DoH 1993) recommended that women should be able to make choices about childbirth, including where their babies are born. This issue of availability of choice does seem to be related to geographical location, with some areas of the country having greater availability of home birth than others (Birth Choice UK 2003). For example, Hull and East Yorkshire Hospitals NHS Trust has a home birth rate of 1.2 per cent, whilst University Hospital Lewisham, London has a rate of 2.6 per cent (Birth Choice UK 2003). A further consideration for the courts may be the mother's rights under the Human Rights Act 1998; her right 'to respect for . . . private and family life' (Article 8) may well include consideration of the right to a home birth.

At the RCM conference on 2 May 2001, the then Secretary of State for Health, the Right Honourable Alan Milburn MP, used the example of the availability of home birth to illustrate the disparity of choice in maternity services across the country:

> In some areas home births are widely available to women; in others they are not. Our standard must be an end to the lottery in childbirth choices so that women in all parts of the country, not just some, have greater choice including the choice of a home birth.

However, in the 2003 Report of the House of Commons Health Committee it was noted that the Department of Health had done nothing actively to achieve this standard. The health committee made a strong recommendation about the inclusion of home birth targets for midwifery students in order to develop and maintain midwifery skills in offering home birth:

> Rather than perceiving home births as a potential drain on scarce resources we see them as a gateway to promoting normal birth and a spur towards midwifery recruitment and retention. We endorse AIMS' (Association for the Improvement of Maternity Services) recommendation that all trainee midwives should be obliged to attend a minimum of three home births as an essential part of their training. We believe that this would help to tackle prejudice against home births among health professionals. But we also believe it would be beneficial if GPs and consultant obstetricians attended a similar number of home births to give them insights into the process and to provide for a more informed and rational debate. (para. 64)

The Royal College of Midwives Position Paper (2002) on home birth acknowledges that the availability of home birth services varies hugely throughout the UK. Nevertheless, although midwives have a duty to provide care for women they also have a contractual duty to their employers. They would not, therefore, be in breach of their duty of care if they refused a woman's request for a home birth because the employers had decided to withdraw home birth services. On occasions, trusts have temporarily suspended home birth services because of staff shortages. One such example is the Chelsea and Westminster Hospital (House of Commons Health Committee 2003).

Midwives who work for an employer who provides a home birth service should ensure that their skills are current in relation to all aspects of care outside an obstetric unit, which would include management of all obstetric emergencies. As a consequence, when an emergency occurred unexpectedly they would be both confident and competent.

Conclusion

This chapter has aimed to prepare midwives to manage emergencies in the absence of immediate obstetric assistance in accordance with statutory frameworks. The discussion of clinical governance and identification of risk management activities highlighted the importance of individual responsibility, as well as organisational responsibility in preventing adverse outcomes for mothers and their babies. In terms of professional and legal accountability, the midwife must act not only within local clinical guidelines wherever possible but also within the scope practice as defined by the Midwives Rules and Code of Practice (UKCC 1998).

The issue of consent to treatment and a woman's right to a home birth is a complex one, and this highlights the importance of working collaboratively with women and all the members of a multidisciplinary team to ensure the safest outcome. This chapter highlights the importance of midwives knowing their own professional boundaries, maintaining evidence-based practice through lifelong learning, and working in partnership with women to ensure safe childbirth whilst maintaining women's autonomy and choice.

References

Birth Choice UK (2003) (www.birthchoiceuk.com).
Bolam v. Friern Hospital Management Committee [1957] 2 All E.R. 118.
CNST (Clinical Negligence Scheme for Trusts) (2002) *Clinical Risk Management Standards for Maternity Services*. CNST: Bristol.
Dimond B (2002) *Legal Aspects of Midwifery* (2nd edn). Books for Midwives: London.
DoH (Department of Health) (1993) *Changing Childbirth: The Report of the Expert Maternity Group*. HMSO: London.
DoH (Department of Health) (1998) *The NHS White Paper: A First Class Service*. Department of Health: London.

Donoghue v. Stevenson [1932] AC562.

House of Commons Health Committee (2003) *Choice in Maternity Services 9th Report of Session 2002–2003* HC 796. The Stationery Office: London.

Hurwitz B (1995) Clinical Guidelines and the Law, *British Medical Journal* **311**, 1517–18.

Kennedy (1993) Medicine in Society, Now and in the Future. In S Lock (ed), *Eighty Five Not Out. Essays to Honour Sir George Godber.* King Edwards Hospital Fund for London: London.

Maynard v. West Midlands Regional Health Authority [1985] 1 All E.R.635.

Mills D H and von Bolschwing G E (1995) Does Clinical Risk Management Improve the Quality of Health Care? *Clinical Risk* **1**, 171–4.

Murray B R and Zentner J P (adapted by C Howells) (1989) *Nursing Concepts for Health Promotion*: Prentice Hall Englewood Cliffs; NJ.

NICE (National Institute for Clinical Excellence) (2001) *Why Mothers Die 1997–1999; The Confidential Enquiries into Maternal Deaths in the United Kingdom.* NICE: London.

NMC (Nursing and Midwifery Council) (2002a) *Code of Professional Conduct.* NMC: London.

NMC (Nursing and Midwifery Council) (2002b) *Complaints about Professional Conduct.* (Reprint of former UKCC Complaints about Professional Conduct, March 1998). NMC: London.

Nursing and Midwifery Council (2003) Press Statement 8/2003.

R v. Adomako [1995]1 AC 17.

R v. Batemen [1925] 19 Cr App R 8.

RCM (Royal College of Midwives) (2002) *Position Paper 25 Home Birth.* RCM: London.

RCOG (Royal College of Obstetricians and Gynaecologists) (2001) *Clinical Risk Management for Obstetricians and Gynaecologists.* RCOG: London.

RCOG/RCM (Royal College of Obstetricians and Gynaecologists and Royal College of Midwives) (1999) *Towards Safer Childbirth Minimum Standards for the Organisation of Labour Wards.* RCOG: London.

Schloendorff v. society of NY Hospital 105 NE 92 (NY1914).

Sidaway v. Bethlem RHG (1985) 1 All ER 643.

St George's Health Care NHS Trust v. S [1998] 2 FLR 728.

UKCC (United Kingdom Central Council for Nursing, Midwifery and Health Visiting) (1998) *Midwives Rules and Code of Practice.* UKCC: London.

UKCC (United Kingdom Central Council for Nursing, Midwifery and Health Visiting) (2000) *Professional Conduct Annual Report 1999–2000.* UKCC: London.

Whitehouse v. Jordan [1980] 1 All ER 650.

Williams J (1995) A Midwife's View, *Clinical Risk* 1, 175–7.

Wilsher v Essex Area Health Authority (1988) 1 All E.R. 871.

10

Managing Childbirth Emergencies: Pre-registration and Post-registration Educational Needs

Karen Bates and Nicki Young

Introduction

At the point of registration student midwives have been prepared to achieve the national pre-registration end-of-course midwifery competencies (NMC 2002). The competencies include the ability to 'undertake appropriate emergency procedures to meet the health needs of women and babies' (NMC 2002 p. 11). When obstetric emergencies arise, the personnel involved must be prepared to deal with the situation promptly and effectively in whatever context they are working. The response needs to be immediate and ordered.

As the introduction to the book explained, the focus is upon the management of obstetric emergencies outside the consultant obstetric unit. Although midwifery training programmes have clinical placements in the community setting, not all students will gain experience of being involved with emergencies outside the hospital environment. However at the point of registration the student is assumed to be fit for purpose and practice, wherever that practice may be.

The chapter on risk and legal management explained that the report of the House of Commons Health Committee (2003) made a strong recommendation about the inclusion of home birth targets for midwifery students in order to develop and maintain midwifery skills in offering home birth. This will allow the students to experience midwives working autonomously away from an obstetric unit, but still does not address the problematic issue of them gaining experience in dealing with emergencies in the absence of medical aid.

The complex nature of the skills that a student midwife must master over a relatively short period of time, requires innovative educational strategies which harness the essence of the philosophy of the profession as well as the unique characteristics of the adult learner (Jarvis 1985). Schools of midwifery have an obligation, therefore, to ensure that midwifery programmes include training to prepare student midwives to recognise, manage and care for women and babies who experience an emergency, in whatever context that emergency occurs. Midwifery schools also need to provide education at post-registration level to ensure that qualified midwives have the opportunity to maintain competence in this area. In addition to this, midwives who have traditionally worked solely in a community setting now find themselves working within integrated systems of care.

Even in emergency situations, midwives need to use professional judgement and demonstrate high-quality clinical-decision-making skills. Every decision needs to be underpinned by a sound rationale. Obstetric emergencies are by their very nature situations of high tension that require quick thinking and speed of actions. However, they can be made even more complex and uncertain if they occur outside the environment of the hospital.

This chapter discusses the pre-registration and post-registration educational needs associated with the midwife's management of childbirth emergencies and will present the strategy implemented by the midwifery team within the School of Nursing and Midwifery at the University of East Anglia to address these. Clinical decision-making surrounding childbirth emergencies will be discussed in relation to novice and expert practice. The discussion will highlight the complexity and uncertainty of this area of midwifery practice when it occurs outside the hospital environment.

The structure of the pre-registration workshops

The theory content relating to the emergencies is delivered across the pre-registration programmes within an enquiry-based learning (EBL) philosophy. The School of Nursing and Midwifery delivers education via the principles of EBL through a mixture of student exploration of clinical scenarios and fixed resource sessions. Great emphasis is placed upon the process of learning and the nature of educational experiences, which encourages learners to be independent and to develop critical thinking and problem-solving techniques (Creedy et al. 1994, Engel 1992, Thomas et al. 1999).

As part of the student preparation for practice and to prepare them for the summative verbal examination, two full-day emergency workshops are held. The workshops build on the knowledge already gained, and allow the student to explore current principles which underpin practice and apply them to the management of obstetric emergencies. The emergencies are usually contextualised in a situation where, for whatever reason, there is no medical assistance available and the student is expected to manage the situation on her/his own until help arrives. It is reasonable to say that medical aid will not be available and the student usually finds herself/himself dealing with the situation in its entirety.

The first workshop focuses upon the emergencies such as shoulder dystocia, breech delivery and neonatal resuscitation which lend themselves to being simulated with the use of dolls and mannequins in the skills laboratory environment. Each student will be guided in the 'hands-on' practice of techniques to resolve the emergency situation.

The second emergency workshop focuses on the other emergencies through a variety of techniques. Scenarios are created which reflect real-life emergency situations. Students work in small groups of three to four and are placed in the role of the midwife to explore how to resolve the situation and formulate action plans to manage the emergency. Following this, individual students have a one-to-one session with a midwifery lecturer, the aim of which is to encourage the student to verbalise her or his management of a specific emergency scenario. The workshops provide the opportunity for students to practise 'emergency drills' and to verbalise action plans in the safe environment of the classroom or skills laboratory.

During the emergency scenario workshops, students are encouraged to verbalise what they are doing and why they are doing it. Authors such as Thiele et al. (1991) and Benner (1984) suggest that this is an opportunity for students to learn decision-making by considering what their responses and actions would be. Simulations of emergency situations may also act as a link between theory and actual clinical practice (Thiele et al. 1991).

Within the pre-registration midwifery programmes the management of obstetric emergencies is summatively assessed by a verbal examination. The use of the verbal examination is the final phase of an on-going strategy within the programmes which aims to assess the students' ability to apply knowledge and understanding to dynamic, complex practice situations and to demonstrate relevant clinical-decision-making skills.

Post-registration education needs

Midwives play a pivotal role in the assessment and management of maternal and neonatal complications. Incorporated in this is the knowledge and recognition of the differential diagnosis and the implications for management in order to reduce maternal and perinatal morbidity and mortality. The central aim of post-registration programmes of education in this area of practice is to enable further development of existing knowledge and skills in a way that reflects the principles of a holistic approach to the care of the woman and the neonate. Within the authors' school, emergency scenario workshops were developed along similar lines to those documented above. They were well attended and evaluated very successfully. These workshops have been superseded by a unit which provides academic credit towards the B.Sc. (Hons) Midwifery Practice pathway and it develops the knowledge underpinning the midwife's clinical skills and actions. It is hoped that these programmes will advance professional practice through the revision and enhancement of the skills and knowledge which midwives already have in relation to this area of practice. As a result, clinical decisions can be justified by the application of critical analysis and synthesis of factual, experiential and intuitive knowledge, as demanded of the proficient practitioner.

The midwives undertaking this unit are required critically to analyse the biosciences which underpin the emergency scenarios and the relevant research literature underpinning the evidence base for management of emergencies during childbearing. This includes not only the physiological sciences but also the psychological effects on the woman and her family. They are required to demonstrate theoretical application to a specific emergency situation of a midwifery-managed case through simulation. Legal and ethical conceptual frameworks underpinning the practice of the midwife in relation to emergency management of childbearing emergencies is also a component of the unit.

It is hoped that these education programmes within the school will inform the clinical 'fire drills' sessions organised locally within the trusts. The Confidential Enquiry into Maternal Deaths (NICE 2001), Confidential Enquiry into Stillbirths and Deaths in Infancy (CESDI 2001), the Clinical Negligence Scheme for Trusts (CNST (2002)) and the Royal College of Obstetricians and Gynaecologists Royal College of Midwives (RCOG/RCM 1999) have all called for the implementation of regular 'fire drills' within the clinical settings so that procedures and protocols can be tested for their robustness, as well as enabling the whole multiprofessional team to work together.

Emergencies within the relative safety of the classroom

Only learners themselves can learn, and only they can reflect on their own experiences (Boud et al. 1985). By encouraging student midwives to examine their own practice and knowledge of emergency situations within the 'relative' safety of the classroom, without fear of 'messing up' in a real-life situation (Race and Brown 1998), the process of reflection can begin. In an effort to make the management of obstetric emergencies visible throughout the pre-registration programmes, we developed teaching and learning strategies to support this very important area of midwifery practice. Post-registration workshops follow this principle through in emergency scenario workshops where midwives are able to examine their pre-existing knowledge and act out their own action plans. Throughout the course of the emergency scenario workshops, it has become clear that there are a substantial number of midwives attending who value the opportunity to act out the processes for managing many of the emergency situations they may well not have been called on to manage in their clinical areas.

The teaching and learning strategy not only prepares the student for practice, but culminates in a verbal examination in the final unit of the programme. A verbal format was chosen for the assessment, as it allows questioning to take place to check the students' knowledge and understanding of the selected emergency. Careful questioning can establish ownership of evidence and allows the student to demonstrate a rationale for all actions.

In the development of the teaching and learning strategy for the emergency situations, the nature of student practice was considered. Studies focusing upon the development of nurses found that novice professionals tend to govern their practice with rule-oriented behaviour (Benner 1982, Benner et al. 1996). Since novices have little experience of real-life emergency situations, they must rely on the rules they have learnt during their training to function. The overall aim of preparing students to manage obstetric emergencies (in the absence of medical aid) is to facilitate their learning of the rules and principles that underpin the management of emergency situations.

Not only must students learn the principles underpinning the midwifery management of emergency situations, they must also be able to explain the rationale behind their decisions and actions. Teaching strategies that combine simulations of clinical situations and thinking aloud techniques may help facilitate decision-making in students (Cioffi 1997, p. 20). According to Scott (2000), the tutor is crucial in facilitating the development of reasoning skills in medical trainees. Tutors can be effective in their role if they insist that both students and tutors make their reasoning processes transparent by thinking out loud.

Decision-making in situations of uncertainty

When obstetric emergencies arise, the personnel involved must be prepared to deal with the situation promptly and effectively in whatever context they are working. The response needs to be immediate and carried out in a systematic order. Not only must health professionals manage the situation effectively, they need to explain and support their actions. Assessment, judgement, and decision-making are all core activities of health professionals, and even in an emergency situation the midwife needs to provide a rationale underpinning all actions.

Carnevali et al. (1984) identified a number of phases in the reasoning processes of health professionals. These include:

* collection of clinical data or cues;
* formulating possible hypotheses;
* weighting of information and interpretation of cues;

- evaluation or judgement of states and conditions to form a mental representation of the problem;
- selection of a decision or set of actions to resolve the problem.

Although appropriate decision-making is expected of all health professionals in all contexts, many decisions are complex in nature and are often made in conditions of uncertainty (Thompson and Dowding 2002). Complex situations involve not only physical cues from part of a patient's presentation but also social, emotional and environmental stimuli (Hayes and Adams 2000) from which health professionals need to discriminate and select in order to reach an appropriate decision (Carnevali et al. 1984). In an emergency this has to be undertaken rapidly and in a systematic order for effective management of the situation.

Many decisions in health care are made in conditions of uncertainty. Thompson and Dowding (2002 p. 15) define uncertainty as 'The inability to predict with accuracy what is going to happen . . . you do not know precisely what the result of your judgement or decision will be.'

Many obstetric emergencies are uncommon and even less frequently met outside the hospital environment. If a practitioner has never encountered a particular obstetric emergency before and the first time they do is in the community setting it may add to the uncertainty of the situation and decision-making.

Community midwives and paramedics face a different set of problems from their counterparts working in a consultant obstetric unit. Community midwives may be the lead professional in a woman's care and are often lone workers attending women in their own homes with limited resources and equipment. Although births at home are usually attended by two midwives, the situation may arise where a community midwife finds herself working on her own until the second midwife or health care assistant arrives. She may be alone when the emergency occurs. Paramedics may well be on the scene prior to the arrival of the community midwife. Working outside the controlled environment of the hospital may lead to situations of even more complexity and uncertainty. Midwives are encouraged to engage with obstetric emergencies by participating in practice drills, which allow the opportunity to apply a prepared action plan to remedy the situation. To a certain extent, the more a practitioner has been able to participate in practice drills the more they will have a sense of what the result of their clinical decisions may be, thus reducing the condition of uncertainty and improving decision-making processes.

Depending upon the length of time as a qualified practitioner, community midwives will have a range and depth of clinical experience to draw from. This may assist them when they are faced with complex and uncertain situations. As practitioners gain domain-specific knowledge and experience in professional practice, they develop the ability to recognise patterns in clinical situations. Pattern recognition has been identified as one approach used by experts when making clinical decisions. Some element of the problem or client triggers memory recall of a similar situation (Coderre et al. 2003, Crabtree 1998). This pattern recognition goes beyond the theoretical and applies to the uncertainty of real-life situations.

In their own domain, experts also develop a sense of salience, which is the ability to determine what is significant for that particular client in a particular situation. They are able to do this by rapidly sorting weighting and interpreting cues to identify meanings. In contrast to the novice, they are able to apply these processes more rapidly without wasting time on possible problem situations which are of less significance (Benner et al. 1996, Biotti and Reeve 2003, Thiele et al. 1991).

However, expertise does not simply equate to the length of time a practitioner has been qualified and working in practice (Benner et al. 1996). Hoffman et al. (2004 p. 59), although writing within a nursing domain, comment that 'expertise is also the incorporation of new knowledge with experience to develop further skills'. One way that health care practitioners can integrate new knowledge with experience is to use reflective techniques. This will facilitate continuous examination and evaluation of practice.

Reflection on the classroom experiences

Kemmis (1985) argues that when a person reflects, they look inwardly at their thoughts and thought processes and outwardly at the situation they are in. By encouraging students to act out their action plans in a classroom situation, they are given the opportunity to consolidate theory learned with practical application. These two processes are given relevance and meaning. By attempting to give theory a contextual setting, it becomes more than a one-dimensional academic exercise in which the dynamic between thought processes, theory and action are lost. However, simulating the experiences also enables students to attend to the feelings evoked when an emergency is unfolding in front of them, in other words, dealing with the adrenaline rush. By providing the opportunity for students to begin to recognise this feeling and deal with the resultant effect – fast pulse rate, dry mouth and a desire to run – will mean that a student is able to adapt her/his management decisions as she/he returns to the experience in a real-life emergency. This same rationale is followed through to the workshops for the qualified midwives.

Conclusion

This chapter has explored pre- and post-registration education needs in the management of obstetric emergencies when they occur in the absence of immediate medical aid. Preparation is via theory and emergency workshops. These workshops use simulations and clinical scenarios to provide the opportunity for examination of practice and development of decision-making skills. They also provide the opportunity for learners to analyse their own uncertainties in a safe and collaborative context. The opportunity to practice techniques to resolve emergencies and to formulate action plans may go some way to decreasing uncertainty in emergency situations. The chapter has highlighted the need for practitioners continuously to monitor their practice as a means of maintaining competence in the management of obstetric emergencies.

References

Benner P (1982) From Novice to Expert, *American Journal of Nursing* **82**, 402–7.

Benner P (1984) *From Novice to Expert Excellence and Power in Clinical Nursing Practice.* Addison-Wesley: Menlo Park, CA.

Benner P, Tanner C and Chesla A (1996) *Expertise in Nursing Practice Caring, Clinical Judgment, and Ethics.* Springer Publishing Company: New York.

Biotti M and Reeve R (2003) Role of Knowledge and Ability in Student Nurses Clinical Decision-Making, *Nursing & Health Sciences* **5**, 39–49.

Boud D, Keogh, R and Walker D (eds) (1985) *Reflection: Turning Experience into Learning.* Kogan Page: London.

Carnevali D, Mitchell P, Woods N and Tanner C (1984) *Diagnostic Reasoning in Nursing.* Lippincott: Philadelphia, PA.

CESDI (*Confidential Enquiry into Stillbirths and Deaths in Infancy*) (2001) *8th Annual Report*. Maternal & Child Health Consortium: London.

Cioffi J (1997) Education for Clinical Decision Making in Midwifery Practice, *Midwifery* **26**, 18–22.

CNST (Clinical Negligence Scheme for Trusts) (2002) *Clinical Risk Management Standards for Maternity Services*. NHS Litigation Authority: London.

Coderre S, Mandin H, Harasym P and Fick G (2003) Diagnostic Reasoning Strategies and Diagnostic Success, *Medical Education* **37**, 695–703.

Crabtree M (1998) Images of Reasoning: A Literature Review, *Australian Occupational Therapy Journal* **45**, 113–123.

Creedy D, Horsfall J and Hand B (1994) Problem Based Learning in Nurse Education: An Australian View, *Journal of Advance Nursing* **17**, 727–33.

Engel C (1992) Problem Based Learning, *British Journal of Hospital Medicine* **48**, 6325–9.

Hayes B and Adams R (2000) Parallels Between Clinical Reasoning and Categorisation. In J Higgs and M Jones (eds), *Clinical Reasoning in the Health Professions*. Butterworth Heinemann: Oxford.

Hoffman K, Donoghue J and Duffield C (2004) Decision-Making in Clinical Nursing: Investigating Contributing Factors, *Journal of Advanced Nursing* **45** (1), 53–62.

House of Commons Health Committee (2003) *Choice in Maternity Services Ninth Report of Session 2002–2003* HC 796. The Stationery Office: London.

Jarvis P (1985) *The Sociology of Adult and Continuing Education*. Croom Helm: London.

Kemmis S (1985) Action Research and the Process of Reflection. Ch.10 in D Boud, R Keogh and D Walker (eds), *Reflection: Turning Experience into Learning*. Kogan Page: London.

NICE (National Institute for Clinical Excellence) (2001*) Why Mothers Die 1997–1999; The Confidential Enquiries into Maternal Deaths in the United Kingdom* Royal College Obstetricians and Gynaecology Press: London.

NMC (Nursing and Midwifery Council) (2002) *Requirements for Pre-registration Midwifery Programmes*. Nursing and Midwifery Council: London.

Race P and Brown S (1998) *The Lecturers Toolkit*. Kogan Page: London.

RCOG/RCM (Royal College of Obstetricians and Gynaecologists/Royal College of Midwives) Joint Working Party Report (1999) *Towards Safer Childbirth: Minimum Standards for the Organization of Labour Wards*. RCOG Press: London.

Scott I (2000) Teaching Clinical Reasoning: A Case-Based Approach. In J Higgs, and M Jones (eds), *Clinical Reasoning in the Health Professions*. Butterworth Heinemann: Oxford.

Thiele J, Holloway J, Murphy D, Pendarvis J and Stucky M (1991) Perceived and Actual Division Making by Novice Baccalaureate Students; *Western Journal of Nursing Research* **13** (5), 616–26.

Thomas B G and Cooke P (1999) Triggering Learning in Midwifery, *The Practising Midwife* **2** (5), 32–4.

Thompson C and Dowding D (2002) Decision Making and Judgement in Nursing: An Introduction. In C Thompson and D Dowding (eds), *Clinical Decision Making and Judgement in Nursing*. Churchill Livingstone: Edinburgh.

11

Improving Working Partnership through Interprofessional Education

Vivien Woodward

Introduction

The increase in community-based, midwifery-led maternity care has reduced medical surveillance of 'low risk' women during both pregnancy and labour. This places a greater onus on midwives, in both emergency and day-to-day situations, to recognise complications and co-ordinate the care and expertise of other professionals, including obstetricians, general practitioners (GPs) and social workers. If women are to have their health care needs met effectively, the development of efficient referrals systems operating in a spirit of interprofessional coalition and co-operation is critical. This chapter identifies evidence which suggests that midwives' referral for assistance in the event of complications is suboptimal and that tensions between them and medical staff are implicated. Interprofessional education (IPE) is identified as a potential process to achieve collaborative working practice and, although this opportunity must be grasped, the lack of a shared vision for maternity care and of mutual trust represents a major challenge.

Referral and communication problems

There is evidence that poor interprofessional relationships currently impact on both women's confidence in and satisfaction with the maternity

207

service (DoH 1998a) and on clinical outcomes. The principal cause of substandard care identified in the Confidential Enquiries into Maternal Death Report (CEMD) (NICE 2001) was ineffective liaison between professionals, and midwives along with other maternity service workers came under criticism. Whilst good practice was commended, midwives' poor communication and teamwork contributed to some cases of maternal death. The report identified that vital treatment for women experiencing complications was delayed owing to midwives' reticence in involving more senior staff, including obstetricians, a problem previously identified in the Confidential Enquiry into Stillbirths and Deaths in Infancy (CESDI 1997). Midwives were also criticised for failing to report complications directly to GPs and other care providers such as the community psychiatric services. The CEMD concluded that midwives lacked a commitment to develop working partnerships, failed to recognise themselves as team members and were diffident about confering with medical colleagues, particularly senior staff. Similar concerns were expressed in relation to midwives' contribution to the NHS Plan (DoH 2003a). The document counselled that midwives can no longer 'go it alone' and need to recognise, respect and utilise the expertise and contribution of others in order for women and families to receive optimum care.

At a time when the increase in community-based maternity care makes effective partnership more essential than ever, interprofessional discord appears to be seriously affecting clinical standards of care. It is essential that these professional differences be settled, and the remainder of the chapter explores the benefits and challenges of interprofessional education as one possible way forward.

The potential of interprofessional education (IPE) to promote collaborative working practice

Effective interprofessional working involves four principles: shared vision, good communication, role understanding and role valuing (Onyett et al. 1996, cited in Miller et al. 1999). Shared learning provides the strategy for establishing these values and improving collaborative working within the maternity services (Smith and Alexander 1999, DoH 1998a). It is important to recognise that shared learning is a general term and needs to be strategically designed and focused if it is effectively to improve interprofessional partnership. It is therefore essential to distinguish interprofessional education (IPE) from multiprofessional education (MPE). IPE involves two or more professional groups who learn from and about one another with the aim of promoting collaborative practice (CAIPE 1997) and often involves client/patient-focused, interactive activities based on clinical cases or scenarios. The approach compares with MPE in which professionals might learn side by side for whatever reason.

Currently, there are IPE initiatives at both pre- and post-registration level, including the NHS-funded New Generation Project, being piloted in the UK, which involves a common learning programme for all health and social care professionals (University of Southampton 2003). The government's modernisation programme identifies IPE as an educational strategy for underpinning its goals for the improved quality of care. For example, the National Plan (DoH 2000) requires the development of working relationships within and between NHS and social care and other non-NHS employers. National Service Frameworks (DoH 1998b) involve integrated care pathways which cross the boundaries between professions and organisations. IPE is already showing promise in nurturing collaborative practice within the context of cancer care and mental health services (NHS Executive South West and Bournemouth University 2000). Whilst IPE initiatives within the maternity services have been limited (DoH 1998a, Smith and Alexander 1999), it is hoped that the awaited guidelines for the maternity strand of the NSF for Children's Services (DoH 2003b) will provide an interprofessional focus and stimulate new maternity services related to IPE programmes.

Nonetheless, as previously identified, referral and communication difficulties reflect existing tensions between midwives and medical staff and the challenge in aligning disparate perspectives and resolving status issues in order to facilitate effective IPE are now examined.

A lack of consensus regarding safety, risk and evidence

Ross and Southgate (2000) identify that whilst it is important that professions maintain their unique identity and distinctiveness they also need to recognise and value interdependence in providing a shared vision of quality health care. Although there are long-standing tensions and rivalries between midwives and medical staff, exacerbated by the medicalisation and centralisation of childbirth in obstetric consultant units (Porter 1995), recent opportunities for midwives to undertake the lead profes sional role, shape midwifery practice and increase community-based intrapartum care appear to have polarised visions of practice even further. Arguably, perspectives could hardly be more at odds, with the midwifery movement promoting normality on the one hand and high levels of Caesarean section suggesting escalating medicalisation on the other.

Midwives and obstetricians might start to develop shared goals where there is an apparent convergence of professional values, and both the midwifery (social) and medical models of maternity care (Bryar 1995) identify the safety of mother and baby as a key principle. However, concerns about safety and the different meanings given to the concept appear to be at the centre of current professional dishar-mony.

The increased scope of midwifery practice and self-governance have required a period of adjustment during which time midwives have had to reskill and strengthen their clinical-reasoning and deci-sion-making capabilities previously eroded by medicalisation (SNMAC 1998). The implications of this change in midwifery status for the medical profession and their central endeavour to preserve perinatal and maternal safety have been expressed as concerns regarding the ability of midwives to provide optimum care. A study was commis-sioned by the English National Board for Nursing, Midwifery and Health Visiting (ENB) to assess the educational needs of midwives to undertake the lead professional role in community-based care (Pope et al. 1996). One-third of registrars participating in the survey (91 in all) thought that midwives were not capable of taking full responsibility for women antenatally and during labour, and expressed concerns regard-ing safety in the event of complications occurring. Of 164 GP partici-pants, some thought that midwives would not be competent to deal with emergencies. This latter finding is also reflected in small studies which have reported the negative attitudes of GPs towards home birth (Hosein 1998, Floyd 1995, Galloway 1995). That many have refused to take responsibility for home births or even to provide emergency cover illustrates the polarisation of opinion between midwives and GPs on the home birth issue.

The topic of home birth perhaps encapsulates the opposing perspec-tives between midwives and medical staff regarding the concept of risk and what constitutes a positive childbirth outcome (DoH 1998a).

Arguably this ideological divergence is increased further by the current emphasis on evidence-based practice (DoH 1998b). Whilst its moral value in providing research evidence to promote clinically effective treatment and discontinue harmful practice is applauded, the status given to the different sources of evidence creates contention between midwives and doctors. Medicine, as a traditionally science-based profession, places the large randomised controlled trial at the top of the hierarchy of evidence. Page (2000), in promoting 'science and sensitivity' in midwifery practice, contests this by advocating the importance of facilitating women's informed decisions by balancing research evidence with the woman's values and feelings rather than prioritising it. This appears to be a sound ethical position as long as decisions and consent are informed.

Even so, just as it is inappropriate for an emphasis on research evidence to override personal values, it is important for midwives not to overemphasise the normal everydayness of birth at the expense at remaining alert to the possibility of complications and emergencies (Hodnett 2003) and death (Mander 2001, Murphy-Lawless 1998). Mander's (2001) phenomenological study of midwives' experience of maternal death identified that they have difficulties in talking about maternal death for a number of reasons, including feelings of guilt, personal failure, defensiveness and the fear of litigation. She refers to 'an occupational denial' of maternal death and suggests that because midwives are unable to 'contemplate the possibility' they are even less prepared for it (p. 256).

Hodnett's caution urges that practice be informed by multiple perspectives and that specific professional values be accommodated within broader, interprofessional goals.

The need to resolve status issues and achieve effective communication

Effective teamworking involves individual professions holding compatible perceptions of their power relationships and interactions with other professional groups (Freeman et al. 2000). For example, expectations regarding leadership and attitudes towards the value of team members' roles. The midwifery profession has argued for equal status for many years and has accrued substantial responsibility and status since the publication of the *Changing Childbirth* report (DoH 1993). Nonetheless, the reality of this change has yet to be internalised and adjusted to by both midwives and medical staff. Midwives have rejected the medical model but have not yet replaced the long-standing medical reference system with one of their own (Wilkins 2000). That obstetricians still exert authority and a strong influence (Edwards 2000) is implicitly evident in midwifery accounts of practice. For example, Hunt and Symonds (1995 p. 129) refer to the 'agonising' experience of attempting to advocate for women, and Page (2000) refers to the added 'scrutiny' attracted to midwives practising one-to-one midwifery when straying from the usual routines.

Whilst midwives in the past may have resorted to subversive strategies in order to overcome their subordinate position and achieve professional goals (Kirkham 1996), equal status is more likely to be achieved by open confrontation and negotiation regarding midwifery's specific contribution to care and how ideological differences can be overcome in the clinical setting (Freeman et al. 2000). The current goal of developing midwifery leadership (RCM 2000) will undoubtedly contribute to this end.

Nonetheless, the bringing together of midwives and medical staff to discuss practice may pose a major difficulty. The findings of a study, although undertaken at local level, indicate personal barriers which midwives need to overcome in order to develop collaborative practice with obstetricians in particular. McFarlane and Downe (1999) undertook a survey of 88 midwives and 171 GPs to identify training needs in South Derbyshire and also explored attitudes towards shared learning. They found that whilst midwives identified the possibility of learning with paramedics, medical students, senior house officers and social workers, they did not identify senior medical staff (obstetric consultants). This compared with GPs who identified that it would be useful to learn with midwives, obstetricians and health visitors (ranked first, second and third respectively). The researchers suggest that it may be a random finding but thought it of interest given that, whilst midwives claim equal status with senior doctors, they showed no inclination to discuss practice with them. The problem, however, is not one-sided. Another study has identified that the attitudes of the medical profession derived from their culture and education inhibiting their readiness to be involved in shared learning (Miller et al. 1999), and a willingness to collaborate appears necessary on both sides.

The challenges in establishing IPE

IPE is the espoused strategy for professional groups to explore and harmonise visions of practice and develop teamwork and channels of communication. However, as just outlined, the difficulties in constructing a shared vision of maternity care practice, accepting a changed balance of power and overcoming communication difficulties are major hurdles in establishing IPE. Also, the value of IPE lies in its potential impact on practice and it cannot be assumed that practitioners learning together and about each other in an IPE context are working and learning collaboratively in clinical environments (Holland 2002). It is therefore necessary for health and social care organisations to promote the principles of interprofessional collaborative practice.

In addition to ideological issues, there are many practical problems to resolve if IPE is to make collaborative working a reality. For example it may be considered how the geographical distances between schools of medicine, nursing and midwifery and PAMS (Professions Allied with Medicine) may be overcome and what content will be of mutual relevance to participants from diverse professional. Timetabling of shared learning may also be problematic since the structures of the various professional educational programmes are often very diverse (Miller et al. 1999, McFarlane and Downe 1999). Because participative educational methods necessitate small groups and facilitators need preparation to take on the role both in terms of educational strategy and insights into the professional contexts and current issues (Holland 2002), IPE has substantial cost implications (Barr 1998). Also, it has been suggested that owing to financial and attitudinal factors, current IPE pilot schemes may be poorly evaluated and preclude IPE being adopted as a permanent feature in professional education programmes (Ross and Southgate 2000).

Conclusion

Managing childbirth emergencies in community settings requires not only that midwives have the skills to undertake life-saving interventions but also that they can effectively detect complications and refer to medical back-up without delay. Interprofessional disharmony must not be allowed to undermine this fundamental element of care.

Although not without immense challenges, the current government promotion of IPE offers a lifeline to the prospect of effective teamwork within the maternity services and to women and their babies who depend upon efficient referrals systems between professions and agencies. This chapter has identified that IPE requires a major cultural shift, at both individual and organisational level, and changes in the delivery of health care and education. This requires the commitment not only of individual professionals to place women and families first and at the centre of care but also of NHS trusts, Workforce Development Confederations and higher education institutions to develop the necessary infrastructure.

References

Barr H (1998) From Multiprofessional to Interprofessional Education. Putting Principles into Practice. In DoH (Department of Health) (1998b) *Learning Together: Professional Education for Maternity Care*. DoH: London.

Bryar R (1995) *Theory for Midwifery Practice*. Macmillan: London.

CAIPE (Centre for the Advancement of Interprofessional Education) (1997) *Interprofessional Education. A Definition*. CAIPE Bulletin No. 13: London.

CESDI (Confidential Enquiry into Stillbirths and Deaths in Infancy) (1997) *4th Annual Report*. Maternal and Child Health Research Consortium: London.

DoH (Department of Health) (1993) *Changing Childbirth. The Report of the Expert Maternity Group. Part One*. HMSO: London.

DoH (Department of Health) (1998a) *Learning Together: Professional Education for Maternity Care*. DoH: London.

DoH (Department of Health) (1998b) *A First Class Service: Quality in the New NHS*. DoH: London.

DoH (Department of Health) (2000) *The NHS Plan. A Plan for Investment, a Plan for Reform*. DoH: London.

DoH (Department of Health) (2003a) *Delivering the Best: Midwives Contribution to the NHS Plan*. DoH: London.

DoH (Department of Health) (2003b) Http://www.doh.gov.uk/nsf/children/ewgmaternity.htm Accessed 19/9/03.

Edwards (2000) Women Planning Homebirths: Their Own Views of Their Relationships with Midwives. In M Kirkham (ed), *The Midwife-Mother Relationship*. Macmillan: London.

Floyd L (1995) Community Midwives' Views and Experiences of Home Birth, *Midwifery* **11**, 3–10.

Freeman M, Miller C and Ross N (2000) The Impact of Individual Philosophies of Team Work on Multi-Professional Practice and the Implications for Education, *Journal Of Interprofessional Care* **14** (3) 237–47.

Galloway M (1995) GPs and Midwives Still Divided on Home Births, *Modern Midwife* July, 7–9.

Hodnett E D (2003) Home-like versus Conventional Institutional Settings for Birth (Cochrane Review). In *The Cochrane Library*, Issue 3. Update Software: Oxford.

Holland K (2002) Inter-professional Education and Practice: The Role of the Teacher/Facilitator, *Nurse Education in Practice* **2**, 221–2.

Hosein M (1998) Home Birth: Is it a Real Option?, *British Journal of Midwifery* **6** (6), 370–3.

Hunt S C and Symonds A (1995) *The Social Meaning of Midwifery*. Macmillan Press Ltd: Basingstoke.

Kirkham M (1996) Professionalization Past and Present. With Women or With the Powers that Be? In D Kroll (ed), *Midwifery Care for the Future. Meeting the Challenge*. Baillière Tindall: London.

Mander R (2001) The Midwife's Ultimate Paradox: A UK-based Study of the Death of a Mother, *Midwifery* **17**, 248–58.

McFarlane S and Downe S (1999) *Southern Derbyshire Training and Education Project for Maternity Services*. Southern Derbyshire Acute Hospital NHS Trust: Derby.

Miller N, Ross N and Freeman M (1999) *Shared Learning and Clinical Teamwork; New Directions in Education for Multiprofessional Practice. Researching Education: Professional Report Series,14*. ENB: London.

Murphy-Lawless J (1998) *Reading Birth and Death. A History of Obstetric Thinking*. Cork University Press: Cork.

NHS Executive South West and Bournemouth University (2000) *Interprofessional Education: Improving Health and Social Care*. Institute of Health and Community Studies, Bournemouth University: Bournemouth.

NICE (National Institute for Clinical Excellence) (2001) *Why Mothers Die 1997–1999; The Confidential Enquiries into Maternal Deaths in the United Kingdom*. Royal College Obstetricians and Gynaecology Press: London.

Page L A (2000) Putting Science and Sensitivity into Practice. Ch. 1 in L A Page (ed), *The New Midwifery: Science and Sensitivity in Practice*. Churchill Livingstone: London.

Pope R, Cooney M, Graham L and Holliday M (1996) *Identification of the Changing Educational Needs of Midwives in Developing New Dimensions of Care in a Variety of Settings and the Development of a Package to Meet these Needs*. English National Board for Nursing, Midwifery and Health Visiting: London.

Porter R (1995) Multidisciplinary Cooperation in Maternity Care. In *The Challenge of Changing Childbirth Midwifery Educational Resource Pack*, Section 3. ENB: London.

RCM (Royal College of Midwives) (2000) *Vision 2000*. RCM: London.

Ross F and Southgate L (2000) Learning Together in Medical and Nursing Training: Aspirations and Activity, *Medical Education*, **34**, 739–43.

Smith L and Alexander J (1999) Educating the Carers. In G Marsh and M Renfrew (eds), Community-Based Maternity Care. Oxford University Press: Oxford.

SNMAC (The Standing Nursing and Midwifery Advisory Committee) (1998) *Midwifery: Delivering Our Future*. DoH: London.

University of Southampton Http://.mhbs.soton.ac.uk/newgeneration/accessed 20/8/03.

Wilkins R (2000) Poor Relations: The Paucity of the Professional Paradigm in M Kirkham (ed), *The Midwife-Mother Relationship*. Macmillan: London.

Index